The Crowning Secrets of Beauty Queens

JAYSHREE PATHAK

JAICO PUBLISHING HOUSE

Ahmedabad Bangalore Bhopal Bhubaneswar Chennai
Delhi Hyderabad Kolkata Lucknow Mumbai

Published by Jaico Publishing House
A-2 Jash Chambers, 7-A Sir Phirozshah Mehta Road
Fort, Mumbai - 400 001
jaicopub@jaicobooks.com
www.jaicobooks.com

THE CROWNING SECRETS OF BEAUTY QUEENS
ISBN 81-7992-603-6

First Jaico Impression: 2006
Second Jaico Impression: 2009

Printed by

Contents

Experts/Bibliography

Madhu Sapre:

Madhu Sapre will always remain the girl who almost became Miss Universe. She hoped to make a career in athletics. Daddy's little girl, she had her father's support when she took her first steps into modelling.

Preeti Sapre:

Madhu's mom, Preeti comes from a royal family, her mother being the first woman to be the member of the Regional Congress Committee. She shares her experience and the efforts taken by Madhu.

Vasant Sapre:

Madhu's dad, Mr Sapre, is a businessman and has a stainless steel casting foundry. He was a body builder and an athlete in his young days. In 1950, he was the title-holder of 'Body Beautiful, Bombay', a body building competition.

Sir G. Isaac:

Assistant director, Sports Authority of India.

Mrs. Kala Soni:

Renowned athlete and a trainer, Kala has been active in international events and had participated twice in the 'Veteran Olympics Championship', in Australia and in the USA. She was the winner in the competition that was held in Australia.

Sangeeta Chopra:

Fashion designer and choreographer, Sangeeta has worked with Sangeeta Bijlani, Juhi Chawla, Sonu Walia, Meher Jessia, Madhu

Sapre, Lara Dutta, Yukta Mookhey, Namrata Shirodkar, Aishwarya Rai and Sushmita Sen.

Gautam Rajadhyaksha:

An ace photographer who has clicked over 200 film personalities over the years.

The Femina Miss India Contest: An Overview

Femina Miss India contest is a known event all over the country and has achieved an international recognition.

Sabira Merchant:

Sabira Merchant is an instructor/panelist for Femina Miss India.

Mickey Mehta:

Micky Mehta is one of India's best known fitness experts. A black belt in martial arts, he holds a diploma in nature care and drugless therapy, therapeutic massage, nutrition and dieting.

Dr. Sandesh Mayekar:

An aesthetic and cosmetic dental surgeon, he has been instrumental in helping many a contestant flash a winning smile.

Bharat and Dorris Godambe:

The hair stylist and make-up artist duo, with their experience of 28 and 15 years respectively, are associated with top models and film stars. They are an indispensable part of fashion dos and film glossies.

Namrata Shirodkar:

Now almost retired from active modelling, Namrata was one of the top choices in early 1990s.

Dr. Shrilata Trasi:

Dr. Trasi is a consulting dermatologist and is also on the panel of various organisations, medical centers and hospitals like The Asha Parekh Hospital, Ram Krishna Hospital as also Indian Airlines, Air India and Jet Airways.

Miss Madhuri Nakle:

As a hair stylist, she has been in this profession for 15 years and has helped the contestants look better.

Aishwarya Rai:

Miss India World 1994, Miss World 1994, the girl with aquamarine eyes. In fact, so far the only Indian model to possess such beautiful eye colour.

Ashley Rebello:

Fashion and costume designer par excellence. Ashley first made headlines when he did costumes for a Hollywood film that was being shot in India.

Daboo Ratnani:

Daboo is one of the leading glamour photographers and has shot almost all the leading models and actresses.

Diana Hayden:

Miss India World 1997. She performed a hat trick at the pageant by winning the Miss Photogenic title and the award for Best Beachwear.

Yukta Mookhey:

The typical Mumbai girl carrying off the coveted Miss World title, beat 93 other contestants from around the world.

Aruna Mookhey:

Yukta's mother, Aruna Mookhey conducts workshops on 'Swiss Chalet' grooming for success at Santacruz, Mumbai, which have benefitted over 300 people, including Yukta!

Dr. Rakesh Sinha:

Dr. Rakesh Sinha is a well-known gynaecologist, surgeon and motivator. He conducts workshops with lecture-demonstrations in various organisations as well as in management institutes.

Ramma Bans:

Dietician, beautician, fitness guru. She was the one who promoted beauty through health and has to her credit 10 health clubs over the years.

Priyanka Chopra:

Miss World 2000, Priyanka Chopra was the only Indian in USA to have been selected at state level for the National Opus Honor Choir.

Dr. Aditi Govitrikar - Lakdawala:

Mrs. World 2001, fair, light eyed, model and Doctor who is fit as a mother, too.

Mr. Shakir Shaikh

Mr. Shakir Shaikh is a well-known choreographer who trains the contestants of the beauty pageants.

Miss India Worldwide Pageant:

Miss India Worldwide Pageant is organised by New York-based Indian Festival Committee, a no-profit, voluntary organisation established in 1974.

Melissa Bhagat:

Melissa was Miss Teen Toronto '95 and then Miss India Canada '98. She travels across the world as a role model promoting unity in diversity among the international Indian communities.

Aarti Chhabria:

Miss Millennium, Miss Worldwide '99, Aarti shares her experience generously.

Yana Gupta:

Yana is a beauty queen born and brought up in Czech Republic but settled in India after marriage.

Dynamic Beauty and Personality Development Institute:

It provides courses in beauty and personality development.

Foreword

It is said that "A thing of beauty is a joy forever." Beauty has been a point of appreciation all over the world since times immemorial. It is human nature to be noticed and appreciated and it is not surprising that the fairer sex desires to be beautiful, a source of attention, appreciation and secret envy.

Beauty, fortunately, is no more only about curves. It has now acquired new dimensions and an altogether new definition. Beauty, today, engulfs grace, intelligence, a healthy and toned body, and an unmatched poise.

Beauty without brains is incomplete. India's beauty queens have time and again proved that they are second to none; they have not only had the honour of being Miss India but also Miss Universe, Miss World and they have been successful with the Pageants too. It is no wonder then that every girl dreams and aspires to be the future Miss India and so knowingly or unknowingly happens to follow her favourite beauty queen as her role model.

But following in the footsteps of a beauty queen is not easy. These beautiful women constantly make efforts to develop and groom their inherent charm and sharpen their minds. All this needs a disciplined lifestyle, a strong commitment and correct guidance. The latter is crucial though till date only the few fortunate ones met the right person who could guide them on to the path of success.

This book promises to unwrap all those mysteries, the secret pathways to success, the endless efforts and the hard work that goes into the making of a beauty queen. It provides detailed information about the fashion contests through interviews with leading models, as also their parents to get a better insight into their experiences as well as the grooming consultants. It also provides fashion tips including health care, skin care, eye care, hair care and the make-up by leading professionals. There is exhaustive information on the Femina Miss India, India Worldwide contest as well as Miss Universe and Miss World contests. In short, the book is an endeavour to enlighten the reader with the nitty-gritty of this grooming profession. It has, however, not been written to propel youngsters to participate in these contests.

Jayashree Pathak

Acknowledgements

Many thanks to a lot of eminent personalities, experts from respective fields, who have been interviewed and provided valuable information. The family members of beauty queens too have proved to be of immense help. I express my sincere gratitude to them.

My loving and heartfelt thanks to Mrs. Sunita Joshi, Dr. Ashok Datar, Mr. Sule, Chairman Sony TV Entertainment, Mr. Vaibhav Pathak, Mr. Vinayak Apte and his family, for their active contribution but for which this book could not have been written.

A special thanks to my Publisher Mr. Akash Shah, Mr. R. H. Sharma and the rest of the team at Jaico for making this project happen.

Above all a special thanks to Padmesh Prabhune.

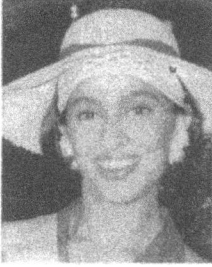

Madhu Sapre – Miss India - 1992, Miss Universe-Runner up

Think about Indian models and one recalls Madhu Sapre, the name that comes to the mind on the spur of the moment. Madhu Sapre is said to be one of the first of the breed of Indian models with international looks. A flawless complexion, fabulous calcium deposits for cheekbones, classic strong features, a 5'8" height and one of the best-kept bodies the fashion industry ever saw.

In fact, one would agree that Madhu Sapre set off professionalism in the Indian fashion industry, till 1992 'The Femina Miss India Contest' was generally a cushy, amateur, low-profile programme, and the winner had to get into the universal arena without any professional guidance, and the only thing she could do was to keep her fingers crossed!

Madhu won the 'Femina Miss India Contest' and was declared Miss India-1992. She was so delighted and touched, that for a moment she could not believe it. "Oh! What a feeling that was!" she says and adds, "It was only when the organisers said that I had made it and within a short time I have to leave for the 'Miss Universe' contest, it sunk in."

Madhu accepted this challenge and was seriously committed to it. She was ready for everything that was considered necessary. How exactly is the contest held? What is the backdrop one needs for it? What sort of questions are likely to be asked...?

Unfortunately, when the time came nobody could really help her in these matters.

Madhu's dad, Mr Vasant Sapre, was very enthusiastic about Madhu's success and worked very hard to dig up every possible information available about the fashion industry and the Miss Universe contest, in particular. He managed to get the videocassettes of the 'Miss Universe' contest which helped her a lot. Madhu learnt many things by just studying those cassettes.

The next step was then to work for a perfect shape and she could think of none other than Mrs. Kala Soni, a family friend, an athlete and a physical trainer. Under her guidance, Madhu was able to reduce her waistline from 26 inches to 23 inches in just 15 days.

Time was running out and Madhu had yet to collect many things. Finally, carrying with her a range of outfits, right from jeans to the National dress, special dresses for rehearsals, the idol of Nataraj presented to her by The Times Group, pairs of payals and, the mandatory evening gown specially designed by Sangeeta Chopra, Madhu flew to Bangkok, the final destination.

On reaching Bangkok, the first thing Madhu did was to offer payals to fellow participants for which she was appreciated. Soon every girl was sporting the *tres* feminine Indian accessory. Madhu had her own way of introducing herself and while handling her visiting card she would always put a bindi on it, surprising most.

Being an athlete and a model, Madhu was sure about her success and having being trained by Mrs. Kala Soni, her spirits were very high. But the moment she saw the tall, 6'1" Miss Venezuela and her exquisite evening gown, Madhu was knocked down for six. She lost her confidence!

"I was crestfallen," she says. "The next thing I did was to go to my room and make a call to my dad saying that I was coming home on the first available flight. All these girls seemed like Hollywood's stars and I felt like Alice in Wonderland. Dad calmed me down and asked me to stay put, not to give up and promised that he, along with my mother, would join me soon. I then relaxed and joined the rehearsal." Madhu further adds, "Surprisingly, I was the one who was nervous but all those girls envied me since they grew fond of Indian outfits."

During the contest Robin Leach, television anchor, posed a question, "Given a chance to change the past, what would they do?" Miss India promptly answered, "Assassination of Mrs. Indira Gandhi as she was one of the greatest leaders India ever had." Madhu was highly applauded by both the jury as well as the audience for her answer. She sailed through the swimsuit round of the Miss Universe contest with a score of 9.9 out of 10 and was adjudged the number one in her Sangeeta Chopra evening gown.

Madhu was now in the final round with Miss Namibia and Miss Columbia. The heat was on. Suddenly a pin-drop silence grasped the auditorium, tension was mounting and all the three contestants could feel butterflies in their stomach.

The judges at the Queen Sirikit National Convention Centre in Bangkok put the final question "What would you do if you were the prime minister of your country?"

Miss Namibia said, "I will work for the cause of children for better tomorrow as they lay the foundation of the future." Miss Columbia said, "I will escort children to the path of peace and love." And in her imperfect English, Miss India Madhu Sapre said, "I would build a sports complex.!" Oh god! Everything was over. She was about to win the title, perhaps, she should have thought out the response for a moment. The answer she gave is probably the most widely discussed and debated.

Even today, Madhu refuses to retract the answer that cost her the crown. "All the officials had told us that our answers had to be truthful," she says, "and had to come from the heart. Nobody told us that we had to be politically correct. I said what I felt and I lost. According to me India has been in poverty for many years, so it was not going to suddenly change in one year by my becoming the prime minister. But there are other areas like art and sports in which we can improve. And being a sports person had suffered, as we don't have the equipment and the grounds in India. In the limited time that we get, to answer, I wanted to say all this but perhaps because of my inadequacy in English, I could not express myself..."

Madhu had come closer to win the elusive Miss Universe crown than any Indian girl and when she returned she drew up a battle plan for the future Miss India: "I told Pradeep Guha of The Times of India to have a swimsuit round for the Miss India competition. He felt that if they had the swimwear round, very few girls would participate. But I urged, 'Then take those girls and have a contest because they will be the best'. I gave in writing how the Miss Universe contest was conducted, and accordingly he prepared for the next contest."

It was this contribution of Madhu Sapre and the willingness of Pradeep Guha to experiment that catapulted the Miss India contest to international standards and eventually won India the Miss Universe crown two years later.

Daddy's little girl, Madhu was brought up in a traditional Maharashtrian family at Vile Parle, a western suburb in Mumbai. Madhu Sapre will always remain the girl who almost became

Miss Universe. Like she will always remain the girl with the Marathi-accented English and faultless, feline body.

She had her father's support when she took her first step into modelling. From then on there's no looking back for her. She has a reputation of being a person who cares little about the world's opinion. 'Her looks can kill' is a comment usually used to describe her. She is a wonderful person with a down-to-earth attitude.

Madhu Sapre set off professionalism and set international standards in the Indian fashion industry the results of which were seen in 1994 - when Miss India turned out to be Miss Universe.

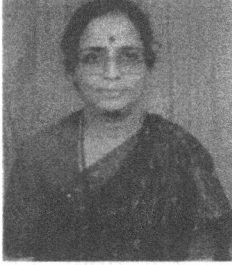

Mrs. Preeti Sapre – Madhu's Mother

Mrs. Preeti Sapre is a typical Maharashtrian lady, clad in a saree with red kumkum on her forehead, hands loaded with green bangles and Mangalsutra around her neck. One look at her and you know where Madhu's chiselled looks have come from. Polite, affectionate and honest, Preeti is a triple graduate and belongs to a royal family.

Meeting Preeti is altogether an experience in itself. She is a bit nostalgic, everything is like telling a story, right from Madhu's school days to her journey towards stardom. She also talks of Madhu's likes and dislikes, her passion for food, especially the delicious Maharashtrian cuisine.

Preeti's mother was a veteran vocalist and Preeti is an adherent fan of Indian classical music. She has also been a radio artist. But the most remarkable thing about her is that she is strongly inclined towards metaphysics and gnosis. Perhaps, she could foresee events when on the day Madhu was about to leave for Bangkok for the contest, Preeti suddenly asked her 'Madhu, what would you do if you were to be the prime minister of India?'

As it happened, Madhu reacted in disgust saying, "Mama... please don't ask anything now, my head will burst." With not much option and not wanting to upset her daughter, Preeti remained tacit and the rest is history!

Once Madhu left for Bangkok, it was very difficult for the duo to kill time. They missed Madhu and decided to go to Bangkok. Both of them would be with Madhu during the practice sessions. After the session Madhu's dad would comment on her performance and, at times, he actually walked on the ramp to demonstrate a more graceful walk!

Madhu was a favourite amongst the girls themselves. They were surprised to see how close she was to her well-knit family. In fact, for some of them, it was something incredible, a father without a girlfriend, a mother without a boyfriend!

Days passed quickly and the countdown began. It was the final rehearsal across the selective audience, just one day before the main show, and it was anticipated that the one who wins during this rehearsal would have the best chance to bag the crown on the final day. Madhu won this crown at the practice session.

Then came the final day. The contest was inaugurated; Madhu succeeded in all the rounds, one after another, and was selected as one of the three finalists. There was a pin-drop silence in the auditorium. The final question was, "What would you do if you were the Prime Minister of your country?" Madhu answered the question and, as every one knows, it was all over! Madhu's dad could foresee the results and his blood pressure shot up. The parents were stunned and speechless.

After the contest, Madhu rushed to her mother and said, "I wish I had taken your question seriously." But the damage was done. Madhu received a prize of Rs two lakh . Had she won the crown, she would have got Rs seven crore!

Madhu's dad thinks that Preeti, instead of asking Madhu a question, should have suggested an answer to the question that she had asked before Madhu left for Bangkok. He himself never asked any questions but always provided her with the information that would help her answer, when confronted with, various questions. Madhu is now an international celebrity and receives a red carpet treatment in Bangkok.

What Madhu's father felt may be valid or not, but Preeti attributes her daughter's healthy, wonderful body to the care she had taken during the time she was pregnant with Madhu. "Never avoid breast feeding the baby; it enhances the power of resistence and makes the child grow up into a healthy individual," she says. Madhu's first ever award was for being a 'Healthy Baby' at the age of three.

A sportsperson at heart Madhu played Kabaddi and Kho-kho in school and was always the one to lead the team. Just before she stepped into college Madhu attended a camp organised by the Sports Authority of India and it was here that she learnt and excelled in running, shot put, discus-throw, long jump, high jump etc. Simultaneously she was also trained in horse riding and swimming. If Madhu were not to be a model, she would definitely have been an athlete!

Mr Sapre, who keenly observed Madhu's progress, decided to encourage her. In fact, it was a 'Project' undertaken unanimously by the family and everybody was assigned their task. Preeti took charge of the business, and Madhu, along with her dad, got busy in the training programme. It was more of a teacher-student re-lationship than a father-daughter one. Madhu won many awards at the state level while in college.

Now that she was to be groomed as an athlete, a training programme was a must. Her body weight was to be maintained at 60 kg. It all started religiously then, the workouts (for 2½ hours), a planned diet that included all types of fruits, vegetables and ghee. Every meal had to be supported with half a lemon and this was a rule that Madhu still follows. The most important thing, however, was the almond powder that was prepared for Madhu which she had before breakfast followed by a cup of milk.

The powder contained 250 gm almonds, one full bowl of sugar, 15 cardamoms and saffron, all slightly roasted. Says Preeti, "Just one teaspoonful of it, followed by milk before breakfast improves the texture of the skin, hair and enhances your vision." The vegetables in Madhu's house were cooked in olive oil and dry chutneys had some sesame oil added to it, again to improve the texture of skin and hair and to better eyesight.

Every thing was going fine. However, to attend her training sessions, Madhu had to miss college lectures but the college was not ready to compromise on the attendance issue.

It's said that things work out automatically if one is destined for it and so it happened for Madhu. She received an offer from another college, Bhavan's college, Andheri, which assured her of readymade notes and a lenient view of her attendance. It also awarded her a monthly scholarship of Rs 1,500.

Now things were working as planned. Madhu also enjoyed her college life. Once during a state-level dance competition Madhu won the first prize with her partner. The chief guests of the function were Garden Vareli's Shah Brothers. Highly impressed by Madhu, they asked her if she would model for them. It was then decided that the Shah's would drop in at her home the next morning at seven and talk to her mom.

Once home, Madhu told her mother all about the proposal. Preeti hated the idea, to put it mildly! But she did not want to be rude and so decided to put lot of unnecessary conditions and to demand more money than it was likely to be offered, all the possible ways of extracting a no from the Shahs. To her surprise, the Shahs accepted every condition put forth by her. In fact, they had come along with the contract papers ready with them.

Preeti handled the professional formalities for Madhu and accompanied her for ad shoots. This ad-endorsement resulted in the record-breaking sales of Garden Vareli and as a result, despite their policy of 'No Repeat Model', Garden Vareli persisted with Madhu for three consecutive ad-campaigns.

The campaign was shot by none other than the ace photographer Gautam Rajadhyaksha. Gautam was bowled over by Madhu's figure and his make-up artist Micky Contractor was so fascinated by her pink cheeks and rosy lips that he suggested that they do away with artificial make-up. Every snap exhibited her beauty. But there was a slight problem. Madhu had a projected tooth. The Sapre's decided to take it seriously. Dentist Dr Karandikar got rid of the little weakness.

Assignments were pouring in. Madhu still managed to pursue her hobby of horse riding, where she met photographer Shantanu Sheoray who urged her to try out rampwalking. Both Shantanu and Gautam Rajadhyaksha met fashion designer and choreographer Sangeeta Chopra who invited Madhu for her next show...

This shift from print modelling to the ramp meant a changed diet. Now the focus was on preferably homemade food, salads, giving up non-vegetarian food, and concentrating on fruit juices, preferably lemon juice. There was an emphasis on tomatoes, cucumber, filtered buttermilk, and a tablet of Seven Seas twice a week, since she had to give up fish. However, quips Preeti, "I had to change Madhu's diet but I continued the almond powder."

Then there were the mandatory multi-vitamin tablets. She battled occasional fatigue with water mixed with lemon, honey and some salt instead of glucose. She always had boiled water and avoided outside food.

Madhu's diet regimen meant:

Morning began with one cup of tea prepared with 1/2 cup of milk, 1/2 cup water, crushed piece of ginger and lemon grass. Lemon grass also acts as a painkiller.

Breakfast was one teaspoon of almond powder followed by one cup of milk, upma or fluffed rice prepared with minimum oil or two pancakes Without oil and then, if needed, a very small cup of coffee made only in milk.

Lunch meant starting off with lots of salads, followed by three chapattis without oil or two bhakris, one bowl of vegetable, half a bowl of boiled sprouted legumes with salt and a very small bowl of rice with dal or curry. Everything would be prepared in minimum olive oil.

Evening snacks were at 4pm where she would have fruits, two biscuits or milk toast with a cup of tea or sometimes a mixture of lemon juice, honey and water with a pinch of salt.

Dinner had to be light. Dal-rice with papad and/or salad but no vegetables for dinner.

Madhu was a successful ramp model and she could deliver her best. She also worked hard on the other angles of her personality. Preeti insisted that she read at least two pages from an English daily and made her listen to English news to improve her accent and diction. This also gave a boost to her self-confidence while interacting with people.

Everything was going well-exercise, horse riding, college and shoots. Once, during a horse-riding practice session, Salman

Khan noticed Madhu and was impressed by her. One day, at his insistence, Helen accompanied Salman to the beach where she exercised, met Madhu and drove her to their house.

Salman's father Salim, a film writer-director, was delighted to meet Madhu and asked her to call up her parents. Madhu spoke to Preeti. The moment Preeti learnt that her daughter was at a filmmaker's house, she lost her temper. Madhu was upset and began crying. It was only when Salim spoke to Preeti, persuaded her and invited the Sapre family for lunch, did she recover. Mr Sapre accepted the invitation, Preeti did not make it. During lunch, Salim proposed a film with Salman and Madhu playing the lead.

"Madhu was just 16 or 17 then," says Preeti. This news spread all over the film industry and Madhu was approached by known personalities from the tinsel town. Once they met her, almost everyone advised her to participate in Femina Miss India contest. It was Sangeeta Chopra and Meher Jessia who got her the application form for Miss India and Madhu, then left with no choice, had to take modelling more seriously than sports.

Mr Sapre encouraged Madhu to participate and win the title. In those days the 'Miss India' contest was a low affair, without any international touch. Daddy's little girl, Madhu, with her father's support ultimately won the 'Miss India 1992' title. From then on, there was no looking back for her.

Madhu is still down to earth and takes special care about small things like avoiding tinned foods. She exercises regularly to keep herself fit and also enjoys swimming. She maintains herself very well and in case you want to know and try it out too, just have a quick dekko at what goes into making Madhu Sapre remain a beauty long after the contest is over:

For Teeth: With great pride Preeti says, "It's hereditary, and we make it a point that all of us have fruits and foods that need to be masticated. As a rule she chews food from both sides of her jaws. She prefers bhakri than chapatti, carrot and radish are her favourites. This provides exercise to the teeth and jaw muscles. She cleans her teeth with Colgate and Pepsodent toothpaste twice, once in the morning and once at night before sleeping. She gargles her mouth after every meal and takes special care of her teeth. As a result she never had to take any treatment like whitening, polishing, etc. She munches roasted rice fluff (chivda) with peanuts and chana dal."

For Hair: The almond powder has helped her a lot, especially her hair, skin and eyes. Once in a week Madhu oils her hair with a gentle massage and washes them the next day with shampoo. Three days later she washes her hair with shikakai. She avoids using hair conditioners. Madhu never has any problems like dandruff. It is only when she has some assignment that she trims her hair and/or goes in for hair perming.

For Skin: Madhu keeps her face clean by washing it with only water four times a day. Once a month she goes in for facial, manicure, pedicure and also applies a face pack of multani mitti. Everyday she cleans her face with cleansing milk and removes artificial eyelids, if used.

Madhu's special tips:

Have a bath twice a day. Use a soap that suits your skin. After bath, apply body moisturiser. Massage your body once in a week, if possible with almond oil. Twice a day apply a hand-and-body lotion. Make sure you eat well and rest at least for eight hours (milk mixed with cardamom and nutmeg helps get sound sleep). Try and avoid late nights. In case of dark circles around the eyes, apply baby oil and massage gently around the eyes before sleeping. Coconut oil on hair before sleeping is also a good idea. Always wash off make-up before going to bed.

For Eyes: Consume almond powder daily and you never have to use spectacles. During facials cover eyes with cloth dipped in rose water. And don't forget to wear sunglasses while outdoors during summer.

For Hands and Legs: Once a month get pedicure and manicure done. Use disposable razors instead of waxing. Use socks to cover the soles. In winter, if needed, apply Nivea's cold cream. Avoid using artificial nails as artificial nails do not allow oxygen to reach original nails and as a result they might deform your original nails. Stick to one particular brand of nail polish that suits you.

Some more: Change your clothes three to four times a day and wash your clothes with Dettol. Cotton clothes suit the Indian climate best. Also use a cotton bed rather than a foam bed.

Mr. Vasant Sapre – Madhu's Father

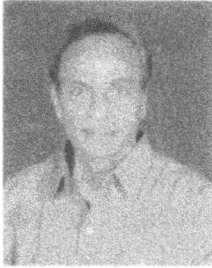

Behind every successful man, there is a woman but in Madhu's case it's the other way around. Mr Sapre is so proud of his daughter that the moment you step into his house he points out to all the mementoes of appreciation of Madhu's achievements. He had wished his daughter to become an athlete but found the world of glamour captivating..

Mr Sapre, a businessman who owns a stainless steel casting foundry, was a body builder and an athlete in his young days and had won prestigious titles.

It was his dream to make her an athlete. He took charge of her training entirely and also taught her weight lifting, sit-ups, aerobics, and free hand exercises. "Fitness exercise is different from sports," he says. "Exercise stretches and relaxes your muscles, keeps your body fit, but to play a game one needs skill. Everyone has a unique body structure and so while selecting a game one should first identify one's strengths and weaknesses."

He also advises reading books on sports and recommends a book called 'The Olympic Book of Sports and Medicine' written by a team of eminent doctors across the world, so as to enlighten oneself on sports in India and abroad. The book provides detailed information on various games and their prospects.

A perfectionist to the core, he was the one who asked and helped Madhu to pen down her experiences during the Miss Universe contest, especially the training one needs for it, which could help future Miss Indias to bag the title, and presented it to Pradeep Guha of The Times of India.

He has been, as Madhu says, "A father who'll be with you, through thick and thin, and through the ups and downs in your life. He'll always be with you when you need him the most."

Sir G Issac – Assistant Director, Sports Authority of India

"Games are to be enjoyed. Be it a cricket match with boundaries knocked all over the ropes or a hockey final with a star player converting the penalty corner into a straight goal.

The Sports Authority of India was formed with a rationale to tap such excellence in sports and so it organises various competitions/tournaments, in the age group of 14-19 years, like the National Championships, National School Games, Grade-A National tournaments, Federation Cup Tournaments and State Championships. The Winners and the Runners-up of these championships are selected and then nurtured over a period of time. Also to enhance their talent they are trained and are further provided with a sports kit, free lodging and boarding, medical care and insurance cover. Once they are through with their training they are introduced in the international arena including the Olympic games. All this is done very methodically. Applications are invited through publishing advertisements in the leading newspapers and circulars are sent to the state and government authorities. Every state has one or two sports training centres. We organise selection camps regularly.

Apart from this the Sports Authority of India has a special 'One Day Boarding scheme' wherein an athlete can attend the special training session and is provided with a sports kit, and a monthly stipend of Rs. 500/- and of course, the exposure to the various competitions and tournaments. The only condition for this scheme is that the athlete should attend his/her training regularly in the morning and in the evening failing which the admission can be cancelled.

Considering the penchant of the general public towards sport and in its efforts to create a 'Health and Fitness awareness' program, the Sports Authority of India has also initiated 'Pay and Play' scheme that is open to the people of all age groups. One can easily register himself/herself by submitting a medical certificate along with the registration form. The activities include athletics, hockey, wrestling, kabaddi and cricket. The fee structure varies according to the various games, and depending upon the game one selects, one has to pay for it."

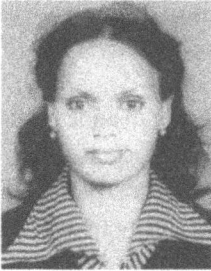

Mrs. Kala Soni – Renowned Athlete and Trainer

"It's very important to have strong muscles to be beautiful and also otherwise, especially back muscles, waist, shoulders and stomach. I am the mother of four daughters and a fitness freak. I am approached for my expertise in long jump, high jump, short put, javelin and discus throw. This is possible because of strong muscles. Normally, after the first delivery a woman's ligaments and muscles lax out, but in my case I could work from the third day, after my delivery, and within a fortnight I was able to carry on with my 'Bent Over' exercises." Kala Soni was instrumental in Madhu's tryst with 'Miss Universe' contest. They started at six every morning and exercised for two hours every day.

Kala Soni's effective tips:

Active in international events and having participated twice in the 'Veteran Olympics Championships' in Australia (where she was a winner) and the US, she suggests some basic exercise for stomach, other than jogging every morning:

Exercises:

1) Stand straight with equal distance between the feet. Stretch your hands in front of you with your fist closed. Hands should be parallel to the ground. Now, without taking any

chair, sit as if you are sitting on a chair. Stretch your upper body vertically upwards while your hands are forward. Count one to eight in your mind and stand up and repeat this at least five times. Gradually, increase the repetitions.

2) Lie down on your back and let your hands lie beside your waist. Lift your knees (as if in a sitting position). Keeping your knees raised up just put your feet down to touch the ground. Now take a deep breath and with the help of the stomach raise your upper body (as if in a sitting position). Do not use your hands. Count one to five and relax and then lie down on your back. Repeat this at least five times. Gradually, increase the repetitions.

3) Lie down on your back, raise your knees up so that your feet touch the ground. Now fold your hands putting palms under your head and let your elbows be in a straight line. Lift your upper body with the help of your tummy muscles and take your head and right shoulder near the left knee. Keep this position till three counts and then relax. Similarly, repeat the exercise this time taking head and left shoulder near the right knee. Repeat the entire exercise five times and gradually increase the repetitions.

4) Take a ball and lie down on your back. Spread your hands in your shoulder line. Stretch your hands at either side. Lift your knees (as if in a sitting position) and hold the ball between your knees making sure that the ankles do not touch. Holding the ball between your knees, bend your legs towards the left side. Repeat the same, this time bend your legs towards the right side. Repeat the whole exercise five times and gradually increase the repetitions.

5) Lie down on your back with your hands spread on your shoulder line and stretch them a bit. Now raise your right

knee so that the right foot touches the ground. Put a ball under the left knee. Taking a deep breath, stomach being straight, try to push the ball away from the waist with your left leg itself. Repeat the same exercise, this time with the left knee raised and the ball under the right knee. Repeat the whole exercise five times and gradually increase the repetitions.

6)   Stand straight, keeping equal distance between your feet and knees straight raise your hands. Now bend forward and touch your toes and relax.

7)   Once you are through with these exercises lie down quietly and relax. Concentrate on your feet and assume that they are slackening off. Cultivate this thought and feel it. Gradually repeat this for every part of your body and let the body relax. Now turn to your left and slowly sit down. Put your right hand on the floor and get up in the bend position and slowly stand straight.

One must exercise daily and push-ups, crunches, squats help a lot. Also to avoid leg injury, one must wear proper shoes while exercising.

Diet: Insist on sprouted legumes, soyabeans, sprouted wheat/ cereals, red rice, paneer, egg, curd (without cream), ample veg- etables like cabbage, tomatoes without seeds, fruits like oranges, lemon, pineapple, etc. Have juice of coriander leaves, as it is very effective for preventing body odour. If possible, have carrot and spinach daily. The proportion of salt, sugar, ghee, oil, condiments, onions and garlic needs to be minimum. Drink lots of water, at least six to eight glasses everyday. Try and have coconut water too.

In case of body ache use pain relieving oil made of half a bowl of almond oil, half a bowl of avocado oil, 1/8 bowl of wheat germ oil, 1 tbsp Rosemary oil, ½ tbsp peppermint and ¾ tbsp lavender. Mix it well to get the homogenous mixture and keep it in a bottle. Shake well before use. Use this oil to massage your body, except your face and feet, in case your body aches after exercise. Apply this at night and you will feel fresh the next morning.

Kala's tips are really useful and we have seen the result in the form of Madhu Sapre.

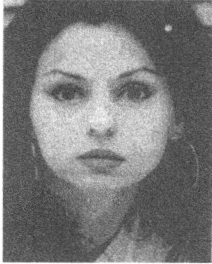

Sangeeta Chopra – Fashion Designer and Choreographer

Daughter of veteran fashion choreographer Shanti Chopra, Sangeeta began her career at the tender age of 16. It so happened that Vimla Patil, then the editor of 'Femina', asked her to choreograph a fashion show and little Sangeeta obliged and her journey on the fashion road began. She was associated with Eve's Weekly Miss India Pageant for a while. Just to upgrade herself and to sharpen her skills, she graduated from The Fashion Institute of Technology, New York.

Ask her about her association with the beauty queens and she quickly says, "Well, both Madhu and Namrata began their work career with me and so I did take them up to the Miss India stage, in the sense they did work a great deal with me before they decided to enter the contest. And I was there with them all the way. Also in the Miss Universe contest, I would rehearse questions and answers with them and preparing what they should be wearing on stage for every function."

Sangeeta has worked with Sangeeta Bijlani, Juhi Chawla, Sonu Walia, Meher Jessia, Madhu Sapre, Lara Dutta, Yukta Mookhey, Namrata Shirodkar, Aishwarya Rai and Sushmita Sen. She adds, "Sushmita has never been in my fashion shows but I designed the wardrobe for her including her winning gown for the Miss India Pageant contest."

Sangeeta's motto is an easy, trendy style. Clothes should be designed in a way that a woman who goes for comfort yet succeeds in being attractive and sexy. She feels that there is always an added advantage to start as a model and then participate in a beauty contest, as you overcome the initial stage fright then. Also one is familiar with walking/posing on stage/ramp and confronting the audience. Namrata, Lara, Madhu, Aishwarya, all were models that turned to beauty contests and their confidence levels were high." She adds, "Earlier on, one could expect special training if you were a beauty queen and then looking on for modelling as a stepping stone. Girls like Meher Jessia, Namrata and alike have done their debut shows with me and I used to train them for one to two weeks but things have changed now. We don't have time to train them for such a long duration. We need quick grasping. The practice for the show goes only for two days before the show and so we work only with professional models or girls who have participated in beauty contests as they are already trained."

Sangeeta feels that the most important thing that any profession demands is the inborn flair, the fire in your belly. The 'Gotta go' approach; only then things work for you. If one has flair then one does not need any training, but if one does not have flair, no matter how much you train her, she can't deliver the best. Stressing her point she says, "Take the case of Madhu Sapre. She is a girl with strong beauty. She doesn't look delicate. Her height, her body, everything shows her strength. She can project herself nicely. It comes out naturally to her. This is the flair, the attitude."

Sangeeta has twice judged the 'Femina Miss India' contest, once for the preliminary round and then for the 'Best Designer Outfit.' She has also choreographed 'Gladrags Super Model' contest, 'Man Hunt' contest and 'Graviera Mr. India' contest. She could make a bid for an entry into the Guinness Book of World

Records. If not, then definitely the Limca Book of Records with 900 shows in her kitty as a choreographer.

As far as clothes are concerned, Sangeeta feels that Indians are followers while our western counterparts are trendsetters. Also fashion is a cycle, "It's like pants. You can wear flats, narrow, straight, ankle length, full length, pedal pusher length, short length. You cannot invent any other form, same is with the fashion; everything goes round in circles. What makes it different is the texture, the fabric you use, the way you accessorise the garment. It's what you mix and how you mix it," she says. "Fashion to me is the way a woman expresses her identity, breaking free from stereotypes and escaping conventions. You don't want your clothes to overpower you", she adds.

Sangeeta Chopra's tips:

Fashion is simplistic and minimal. The future of fashion lies in discrete and distinct. It is advisable to have different sets for office and work and the evening dresses should be separate. For evenings it is always advisable to have mid-lengths or full-lengths with tops. Of course, fashion is still about personal preferences but one should give a thought to it. One should select a dress that suits her and should stick to it.

As for the selection of colour and dress, a short girl should try and wear only one colour from top to bottom instead of wearing two different colours. Dark or brown girls should wear more neutral colours and not very bright colours like, say parrot green or, for that matter, bright blue. Everyone has a certain colour that doesn't suit them. It has nothing to do with one's skin colour. Colour is something that reflects your nature and personality. A shy girl in sober colour like white or cream color seems pretty but she may not look good when dressed in bright colours.

Normally bright colours suit outgoing smart girls. One should choose a dress in which she feels comfortable and confident and not awkward. Also every designer has specific ideas and as fashion changes regularly so does the design. Sangeeta admits, "I personally prefer western outfits but I also design Indian outfits."

Modelling is of two types: Ramp/Stage modelling and Print or Photo modelling. For ramp modelling, one should have a height of at least five ft. six inches to five ft. eight inches. For Print modelling even a height of five ft. two inches would do, if one has a beautiful face. A model has to be slim and good-looking.

For both the types of modelling, striking features are vital. A model with high cheekbones, big eyes and arched eyebrows is captured marvellously in photographs and emerges very beautifully in ramp shows.

A model's hair should be of uniform length and not in steps. It is advisable to have shoulder-length hair so that various hairstyles can be tried according to the costumes. If a model has short hair, she won't look good in an Indian dress and long hair doesn't suit western outfits.

Beauty without brains is of no use. An aspirant should have good general knowledge. Also individuality is a must. Be original, for by copying others nobody can do well.

If you are an aspiring model, here is a final checklist for you:

Check yourself and analyse if you meet the criteria as mentioned above.

Get the portfolio done from a photographer in various costumes and different make-ups and hair-dos. Shoot length, close ups and mid-length.

Take these snaps (mentioning your height and contact numbers) to various ad-agencies, model coordinators and production houses.

Then follow up with them, asking, "Sir, have you seen my portfolio? Could I have the opportunity to work with you?" And you may get a break. Take care that nobody takes you for a ride.

Then it all depends upon your effort and hard work but don't give up, as you will definitely get better opportunities.

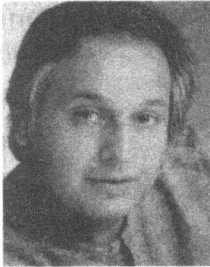

Gautam Rajadhyaksha – Ace Photographer

Converting a hobby into a profession is easy, especially if you are as good at it as Gautam Rajadhyaksha is. The glamour photographer has clicked over 200 film personalities over the years. Since his childhood, Gautam was a Hollywood buff and was always inspired by the portraits of Hollywood stars. Later, while working as the head of the department in photo services, for Lintas Advertising, he had the opportunity to get in touch with legendary photographers like Adrian Steven, Vilas Bhende and Mitter Bedi, and take a shot at the camera.

Gautam began with shooting friends like Tina Munim and Anna Bredmeyer. Says he, "Sometime in 1980, Shabana, Javed and I were spending a lazy Sunday at my place. As the late afternoon sun slanted into the room, I impulsively asked Shabana if she would allow me to shoot her. She was willing. She liked the results and within a month, I got a call from a film monthly asking me to shoot Shabana for them, as she had made a special request for me. In a panic I called her and confessed my total lack of confidence. 'But I am confident,' she said firmly, 'besides if the pictures don't come out well, we'll do them again.' There was no backing out of this one..."

Gautam has done a lot of campaigns on consumer products, soaps, beauty products, cosmetics and alike. He has done series of covers for Femina during the late '80s and early '90s and even now many a times does a cover for Femina. He has done photo shoots for Madhu Sapre, Namrata Shirodkar, Raveena Tandon, Twinkle Khanna, Tejaswini Kolhapure, Amitabh Bachchan, Rekha, Kajol and many others. A photographer plays an important role in the glamour world as he is the one who is going to capture your beauty and present it charismatically. It's his skill, his talent that helps an aspiring model to get through the doorway. He was the judge for the Femina Miss India contest 1992 along with Ashwini Bhave and Sangeeta Bijlani. During the contest it was decided unanimously that if they were to send Miss India abroad then they would select a girl with minimum height of 5'7" for, in the international arena girls have a minimum height of 5'9" to 5'10" and the chances of an Indian girl to make impact holds only if she is of optimum height.

Gautam is very clear when it comes to what constitutes a pho-togenic face and says, "A photogenic face is a very abstract notion and there is nothing called photogenic or non-photogenic face. One may have a very beautiful face and features and still may not get effective photographs, whereas I have seen so many faces that are not conventionally beautiful but they appear so glamorous. This is all about communication, the way one communicates with the camera. It's just projecting oneself in front of the camera and it captivates these features."

According to him, while shooting a portfolio a male model may take anywhere around four to five hours for a photo session whereas a female model may take seven to eight hours, for the time is consumed on various hair-styles, make-up, costumes and so on.

"I have some basic principles", says Gautam. "While doing a shoot for a model photographers must understand one thing that the focus should be on the model and so they should try their skills to make him/her look charismatic than use various techniques.

"I feel sorry to say but I have seen many photographs where techniques like cross-processing, obscular lights and so on actually take away the focus from the object. A photographer should be able to depict a model's features, various reactions and feelings."

"Though it is possible to make a fat person appear slim by asking them to wear dark clothes, the best thing is that they take care of themselves by exercising, having a balanced diet and be confident about themselves. This will not only make the person appear beautiful but also help him/her have a great portfolio. A beautiful and healthy body helps to have an effective portfolio."

Gautam has a message for the aspirants, "Prepare yourself thoroughly before you choose modelling as a career and work on it rather than just hopping in."

Gautam Rajadhyaksha's tips:

Analyse yourself according to the profession. Ask yourself, "Are you fit for this profession?"

Prepare yourself and keep yourself updated about the happenings in the profession like fashion trends, dress designs, photography and realise the need to have an effective portfolio. Get it done according to the current techniques.

Get the portfolio done with due concentration, if needed devote some time (perhaps for body toning, hair care, hair style and alike) to make yourself presentable and then get the shoot done as an effective and expressive portfolio can get you assignments over a longer period and boost your self-confidence.

Don't run after a fashion but select (dress/colour combinations and hair styles) things that suit you. All these efforts help the photographer to be creative and can also enhance the self-confidence of the aspirant.

The Femina Miss India Contest: An overview

Femina Miss India contest is a known event all over the country and has acclaimed an international recognition over the years. Thanks to Madhu Sapre and the management of The Times of India for their quest, zeal and passion towards the fashion industry, we have seen the results now.

Organised by the 'The Times Of India Media Group' the contest ropes in the galaxy of beauty across the country creating huge hoopla. It all started way back in 1947, the Indian Independence year, and was then organised by 'Eves Weekly' as press selection and was later brought under the 'Femina -A Times Group' publication and is now called 'The Times Of India Media Group.'

The winners of Femina Miss India contest are awarded titles like 'Miss India Universe', Runner-up I is awarded the title 'Miss India World' whereas the Second Runner-up is declared as 'Miss India Asia-Pacific'.

Year	2000
Miss India Universe	Lara Dutta
Miss India World	Priyanka Chopra
Miss Asia Pacific	Diya Mirza

Year	1999
Miss India Universe	Gul Panag
Miss India World	Yukta Mookhey
Miss Asia Pacific	Shivangi Parekh

Year	**1998**
Miss India Universe	Laimarina D'Souza
Miss India World	Shweta Jaishankar
Miss Asia Pacific	-------

Year	**1997**
Miss India Universe	Nafisa Joseph
Miss India World	Diana Hayden
Miss Asia Pacific	Divya Chauhan

Year	**1996**
Miss India Universe	Sandhya Chib
Miss India World	Rani Jairaj
Miss Asia Pacific	Mini Menon

Year	**1995**
Miss India Universe	Manpreeet Brar
Miss India World	Preeti Mankotia
Miss Asia Pacific	Ruchira Malhotra

Year	**1994**
Miss India Universe	Sushmita Sen
Miss India World	Aishwarya Rai
Miss Asia Pacific	Shweta Menon

Year	**1993**
Miss India Universe	Namrata Shirodkar
Miss India World	Karminder Kaur
Miss Asia Pacific	Pooja Batra

Year	**1992**
Miss India Universe	Madhu Sapre
Miss India World	Shiela Lapez
Miss Asia Pacific	--------

Year	**1991**
Miss India Universe	--------
Miss India World	Ritu Singh
Miss Asia Pacific	--------

Year	1990
Miss India Universe	Sangeeta Bijlani
Miss India World	--------
Miss Asia Pacific	--------

Year	1989
Miss India Universe	Susan Sablok
Miss India World	Navia Mehndi
Miss Asia Pacific	--------

Year	1988
Miss India Universe	Dolly Minhas
Miss India World	Shikha Swaroop
Miss Asia Pacific	--------

Year	1987
Miss India Universe	Priyadarshini Pradhan
Miss India World	Manisha Kohli
Miss Asia Pacific	Queenie Singh

Year	1986
Miss India Universe	Meher Jessia
Miss India World	Anna Verghese
Miss Asia Pacific	Poonam Gidwani

Year	1985
Miss India Universe	Sonu Walia
Miss India World	Sharon Clerk
Miss Asia Pacific	Vinita Vasan

Year	1984
Miss India Universe	Juhi Chawla
Miss India World	Suchita Kumar
Miss Asia Pacific	Nalanda Bhandari

(The above list also contains winners of the Eves Weekly.)

Eligibility for the contest:

Any individual with an Indian nationality. Must be in the age group of 18-23 years. Having a minimum height of 5'6". Should be unmarried.

Documents desired:

Bio-data

Photographs - Full length, Close up, Left profile and Right profile.

Address: The above documents should be sent across to The National Director, Femina Miss India, 2nd Floor, The Times Of India Bldg, D.N. Road, Mumbai 400 001-India.

Titles:

Miss India Universe, Miss India World, Miss Asia Pacific, Miss 10, Miss Beautiful Smile, Miss Photogenic, Miss Talented.

Selection:

Among the total number of entries received around 29 contestants are short-listed and are then trained for five weeks. Professionals/consultants are hired for various categories.

The contest is categorised into Preliminary rounds and the Main event. The preliminary round involves selection of Miss Beautiful Smile, Miss Photogenic, Miss 10 and Miss Talented. The main event called the 'D-day' is the day of finals and involves selection of Miss India Universe, Miss India World and Miss India Asia Pacific.

While calculating the marks, the highest and the lowest marks obtained by the participant are ignored and the average of the remaining marks is considered as the score. If there is a tie in the final round a common question is asked to the contestants and depending upon the marks the winner is announced. All the contestants are awarded token gifts apart from that winners are awarded prizes and gifts from various reputed companies.

Let's just check it out to get a feel...The Femina Miss India 2000.

The Preliminary round was conducted at Lalit Kala Thoranam, Hyderabad.

The show began with traditional Indian performance and the hosts for the night, Rahul Khanna and Malaika Arora Khan took charge. Cyrus Barucha was present too.

The judges on the panel were film stars Sonali Bendre, Twinkle Khanna, Gulshan Grover, Arjun Rampal, Marc Robinson, Bipasha Basu and Miss India '86 Meher Jessia. Miss World '99 Yukta Mookhey did oblige the host and shared some time on the stage. The names of the contestants were being announced and accordingly models walked through, Priyanka Chopra, Lara Dutta, Diya Mirza...and the others. There were 26 contestants in all. It was like an array of beautiful bodies and minds, fascinating, charming and glorious.

Contestant #14 Diya Mirza was selected as Miss Beautiful Smile, while contestant # 24 Lara Dutta was selected Miss Photogenic. Contestant # 8 Waluscha was selected Miss 10 and contestant # 7 Yogini was selected Miss Talented.

Yukta Mookhey handed over the crown and the coveted belt to the winners.

The main event, Femina Miss India Final was held at Poona Club Ltd., Pune. The evening was full of music and entertainment. Also present were international artists who fascinated the audience. They came from the Caribbean islands and the East European countries. The show began with a troupe dance and the contestants emerged through the lobby wearing their designer costumes. Each of the contestants was introduced with her number and all did their catwalk. Mega stars Shahrukh Khan and Juhi Chawla were among the judges. Designer Jaspreet and Bhavana accepted the award for 'Best Designer and Costume Prize'. There was also the beachwear round which saw only the 15 contestants selected in the first round. Later each of the contestants chose their judge and had their questions. Of these contestants, five finalists were selected depending upon their performance. A common question was put to these finalists "Had you been the Police of the Eden garden whom would you punish? Adam, Eve or the snake?" There was a tie. As a rule it was not disclosed among whom was this tie and so there was the final common question "If it is said that happiness lies in ignorance then why do we struggle for knowledge?" This was answered too. One could feel the excitement even as silence grasped the auditorium.

This was followed by a tribute to the successful models of the 90s and trophies were awarded to Madhu Sapre, Namrata Shirodkar, Manpreet Brar, Divya Chouhan, Ruchita Malhotra, Diya Abraham and Shweta Jayshankar. And then all the 26 contestants paraded on the stage for the last time.

Then came Shivangi Parekh, Yukta Mookhey in her Miss World-winning evening gown and Gul Panag to the stage to hand over the crowns. It went like this...Second Runner-up Diya Mirza!! A huge applause from the audience. First Runner-up Priyanka Chopra!! And the Miss India Universe is ... Lara Dutta!!.

Electrifying and joyous, it was the moment of a lifetime for the three of them, and in particular, for the newly-discovered Lara Dutta.

This is how the Femina Miss India contest happens!

Sabira Merchant – Instructor/Panelist, Femina Miss India

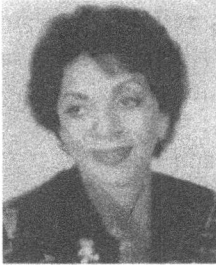

Sabira Merchant conducts courses on speech, diction, public speaking and etiquette. In fact, she has to her credit the task of training several Miss India's on stage presence and public speaking. This is one of the important aspects of fashion contests. There are so many instances like Sandhya Chib Miss India 1996, Madhu Sapre Miss India 1992, Rani Jayraj Miss India World 1996. All these girls made a difference just because of their answers, perhaps they were not trained, but it really matters. This is where Sabira comes and helps them; she educates them on speech, diction, public speaking, stage presence and etiquette. Sabira is associated with the Femina Miss India for quite some time now, and when it comes to training she emphasizes categorically, "You have to give a best shot to see that all the plus points of the candidate are highlighted effectively."

The training consists of 25-30 days, prior to the contest, which includes six lessons of two to three hours each on diction, stage presence and interaction with judges and/or audience. It also includes lessons on table manners, posture, gait and giving the correct response. This is taught by playing video cassettes in order to identify their mistakes and then to correct it accordingly. Of course, the onus lies on the candidate once the training is through. Says Sabira, "I always suggest them to highlight their talent in their own way and never copy someone. Believe in yourself and success will follow you. All of us have our individuality and we should maintain it."

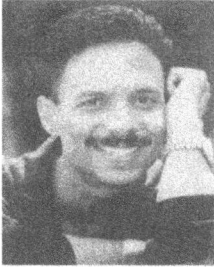

Micky Mehta – Fitness Expert

Micky Mehta is one of India's best known fitness experts. A black belt in martial arts, he holds a diploma in nature care and drugless therapy, therapeutic massage, nutrition and dieting. Over the years he has been a consultant in aerobics, weight management and body sculpting and has produced physically perfect winners like Yukta Mookhey, Diana Hayden, Lara Dutta, Ujwala Raut, Manpreet Brar, Priyanka Chopra, to name some.

Says Mickey, "Attitude, integrity, karma and philosophy form the foundation stone to a perfect human body and the entire personality of the man stands to grow when they are in the right proportion. Also, various forms of energies are present in human beings and in the nature around us, and the process of 'give and take' of these various cosmic and human energies; to polish the above qualities form the basis of spiritual health."

"The concept of exercise is based on the principles of Yoga to gain total fitness. Total fitness is an integration of all your faculties... the physical (that's your body), your mind and your spiritual side...your spirit. Only when all these three together are developed and are harmonious, can a person be positive, happy, creative and confident! When you work out you should do that in such a way that all the glands, the mephitic system, psycho system, muscular system are stimulated properly and also your muscles are toned up. This really gives you energy and you will feel happy and confident."

According to Mickey, the physiological ways to keep oneself clean are through bladder, bowels, skin and exhaling. If any of these channels doesn't function properly then one may have some problems. The best way to be fit is to breathe properly. He goes on to give an example. "To maintain psychological cleanliness we need to breathe properly. When we inhale we take in the vitality, the spiritual radiant, energy, love and peace, and when we exhale we give out all the negative emotions like anger, distrust, hatred etc. Once you realise this you will feel better and over a time your body will respond automatically."

He feels that the spiritual side is often neglected by trainers. "To attain mental calm and spiritual balance it is important to remain silent or meditate for five minutes or so, three to four times daily. Listen to your inner voice and get connected with the universe. Calm yourself for a while during the day and discover a more compassionate and sensitive side of yourself," he says.

As far as diet is concerned, Mickey feels that the colour of the food that you eat is important. Says he, "Deep coloured fruits and vegetables contain more antioxidants than the light coloured ones. For eg. Spinach, carrot, beetroot, pomegranate, grapes, strawberries etc. each of them have their own therapeutic value. Cabbage contains potent antioxidant that prevents breast cancer. It is advisable to have it raw or very lightly cooked. Apart from being good for eyesight, carrots are packed with beta carotene that helps in lowering blood cholesterol. The orange pigments in carrot boost the immune system and increase the body resistance. Having a glass of carrot juice every morning can reduce the risk of cancer even amongst smokers; oranges contain a wide range of antioxidants that help fight cancer and lower cholesterol and blood pressure. As far as grapes go (black grapes are better than green), they have the tendency to prevent blood clots in arteries and so it is always good to have one glass of black grapes' juice. Onions too are full of antioxidants that prevent formation of blood clots in arteries. They also maintain the cholesterol level in the body. They make causative agents for cancer inactive. Spinach cuts the risk of lung cancer, heart disease and cataract. It also has anti-aging ingredients.

Tomatoes contain Lykopen, an antioxidant that prevents cancer of oesophagus, stomach and large intestine. Even if you boil them the level of Lykopen is not disturbed. Hence they should be consumed regularly.

Psychological exercises

Meditation is the best exercise. It gives you mental peace and you will definitely feel better. Sit in a cool and lonely place. Close your eyes and try to concentrate on breathing.

Take a deep breath in. Remember when you breathe in/inhale you take in the vitality, the spirituality radiant, energy, love and peace, and when you exhale you'll give out all the negative emotions like hatred, fear, sense of insecurity etc.

Now while you exhale relax slowly. Let each and every organ of your body relax. Do not bend your back, sit straight. While breathing in fill in positive attitude, while breathing out give out all the negative attitudes. Continue meditating for more sets. Meditate every day, regularly. This cleans your system at a psychological level and once you realize this you will feel better and over a time your body will respond automatically.

Mickey Mehta's training schedule:

Mickey has designed a special 28-days training schedule that helps to lose fat and tone up your body. Also it removes the toxic agents from your body. The 28 days (four weeks) programme is divided into four phases. But he warns that before going in for it one has to keep a few things in mind.

Follow the eating habits as stated. Remember do not look for taste, you cannot have this luxury. Satisfy your hunger not appetite. Food is the basic need of your body.

In case you happen to have a break in between a schedule, start again from day one.

Use rock salt than the table salt.

By adhering to this detox program you will not only feel good but also smell, look, think, behave and perceive good.

Apart from raising immunity levels and improving concentration this program will regulate your menstrual cycle and sort out skin and hair problems.

Water is the core element of this schedule. So whenever you feel thirsty, just pour water into your belly as much as you can but do not drink water unnecessarily.

Meditate regularly. Regulated breathing is very important. While exercising, inhale and exhale properly.

While exercising, take note of every movement in your mind as this helps the body to respond properly and can get the maximum benefits of exercising.

Do not make haste while you exercise. To avoid discomfort or injuries while exercising please go very slow on your breathing and exercise movements.

By following this schedule, you will not only look better but you will also get your body in shape. To get a unique body structure, follow this schedule regularly for 3 months that is continuing this 28-day schedule three times.

It is crucial to do the warm-ups before you start exercise.

Warm up: Stand straight, take a deep breath and move your hands front and back, also move your chin accordingly, that is, raise your chin when your hands are in front and down when your hands are back. Do it 16 times.

Stretch your hands with your palms up and extend it over your head, as far as possible. Keep your chin up straight with your lower back being a bit arched (15 times).

Stretch your hands forward, then along sideways with your chest, shoulders and neck being stretched upright (15 times).

Stand straight, taking a deep breath raise your hands straight and then bend down to touch your toes keeping your knees straight (12 times).

This was the warm-up which is common and has to be done before doing any exercise.

Phase 1 (First week)

During the first week proper care should be taken regarding food habits and the exercise. The workout consists of different exercises that have to be followed after the warm up.

Stand straight. Breathe in and go up. Breathe out and come down. Breathe in and half squat. Breathe out and straighten (12 times)

Put your hands behind the head, take a deep breath, breathe out and move upper body sideways, elbows pointing downwards to your hips. Move first to your right side and then on the left side, your legs being straight and firm. (16 times)

Stand straight and join your hands (as in Namaste position). Keeping your hands in the same position raise them upwards above your head and start spot walking raising your knees as high as possible.

Lie down on your back. Stretch hands behind. Take a deep breath and while breathing out lift your neck, head, shoulders, arms and upper back and then lie down on your back. (12 times). Then lie down, body totally limp and eyes gently shut. Breathe in and out slowly for 3–4 minutes before getting up.

Diet for the first week
Day 1 and 2: Start your day with lemon juice mixed (without adding sugar and salt) in ½ glass of water. This mixture of lemon in water is called Lemon-shot and acts as a detoxification agent. It soothes digestive system, gives energy and helps in digestion, assimilation and excretion.

After some time, say 15 minutes, have a glass of coconut water. Try to consume 3-4 glasses of coconut water in 3-4 hours. The coconut water has to be non-refrigerated, as extreme temperatures are not good for body. Around 11 am have 2 sweet limes and then onwards continue having 2 sweet limes at the interval of every 2 hours. In between have one lemon shot. Just before sleeping have 2 glasses full of coconut water followed (in the 30 min) by a lemon shot.

Day 3: Have 8-10 glasses of coconut water throughout the day and do not forget to consume their tender kernel.

Day 4: Start your day with a lemon shot followed by 3-4 glasses of coconut water over a period of 3 hours. Around 10:30 am have one plateful of sliced fruits, like papaya, mango, apple. For lunch eat a cheese plate full of salad followed by a simple meal of 2 rotis made of jowar, bajra or corn with a bowl of oil free cooked vegetables. 4 hours later have one lemon shot. At around 7:30 pm enjoy a big bowl of fresh tomato soup without any flour. Do not forget to have a lemon shot before sleeping at night.

Day 5: Starting from morning right till the afternoon, have sweet lime or oranges or eat the same every two hours. Have lunch same as of day 4. Four hours later have a lemon shot followed by a bowl full of soup at 7:30 pm in the evening. Have a lemon shot at night before going to bed.

Day 6: Feed yourself with as many water melons as you like, for the day.

Day 7: Start your day with a lemon shot and after an hour, begin drinking 3-4 glasses of coconut water till 11 am. Follow this with 8 dates (the stone fruit, commonly called Khajur) with one cup tender coconut's kernel whenever you feel hungry. During the day try to sip in 2-3 glasses of coconut water, without fail. Have your dinner as per the schedule and before sleeping have the lemon shot.

Phase II (Second Week)

Do the warm up exercise by increasing every count by 8.
Repeat exercise 2 of phase I.

Spot walk slowly with arms moving in circular motion for 2 minutes. For the next 2 minutes continue spot walking with arms opening and closing horizontally. Then continue spot walking with arms stretching up and coming down on your legs slowly for 2 minutes. In all do spot walking for 6 minutes.

Spread your legs with feet double your shoulder width. With one arm behind your back lift the other arm up and stretch to the opposite side horizontally going back and forth (14 times).

Lie down on your back. With your hands stretched behind, take a deep breath and slowly move up and touch your toes, exhaling. Now breathe in and repeat (15 times).

Lie down on your back and just do the Air cycle (10-12 counts). Relax.Air cycle. Relax. Air cycle. Relax.

Diet for the Second Week:

Day 1: Feed yourself with coconut water only as much as possible - whenever thirsty or hungry.

Day 2: Drink coconut water whenever you feel thirsty and have 8 dates (the stone fruit commonly called Khajur) with one-cup of tender coconut's kernel whenever you feel hungry during the day.

Day 3: Start your day with vegetable juice consisting of carrot, beet, cabbage and tomatoes mixed with lemon juice and rock salt. Have this juice over a period of 2 hours. For lunch have 1 bowl full of rice (unpolished) and curry, with salad. 4 hours later have a lemon shot. In the evening have one plate full of sliced apple, pears or guava. Before sleeping have 2-3 glasses of coconut water.

Day 4: Start your day with lemon shot. An hour later eat a plate full of chopped fruits like apple, papaya, banana, chickoo etc. for lunch have a big bowl of medium thick dal garnished with spinach, onion, coriander leaves for lunch. 3 hours later have a lemon shot. After 6 hours of lunch, eat 1 small bowl of seeds and nuts, cashew nuts and so. Do not forget to have coconut water before going to bed.

Day 5: All day eat bananas, as many as you like.

Day 6: Start your day with a lemon shot. Have 3-4 glasses of coconut water over a time of 3-4 hours before you have your lunch. For lunch have 2 bhakris (of jowar/bajra) and 1 bowl full of oil free boiled vegetables or dal, have some salad too. Take a lemon shot after 4 hours of your lunch. In the evening have a big bowl of grated potato and spinach soup. 3 hours later drink 2-3 glasses of coconut water before sleeping at night.

Day 7: Start your day with a lemon shot. After an hour, follow it with a bowl full of sliced/grated carrot. In the afternoon have a big bowl of chopped tomato and cucumber. In the evening eat a bowl of grated carrots. For dinner again eat a bowl of chopped tomato and cucumber. Have a lemon shot at night and go to bed.

Phase III (Third Week)

Repeat warm up exercise and increase each exercise by 10 counts.

Spot jog slowly with arms circling back and forth, inhaling and exhaling very slowly for 2 minutes. For the next 2 minutes continue spot jogging, with your arms opening and closing horizontally. The next two minutes spot jog with arms moving vertically. Now spot walk for 3 minutes to slow down.

Take a stick/rod and hold it behind your neck. Twist your upper body gently backwards slowly and then come to the original position. Breathe out when you twist and breathe in when you come to the original position (16 times). Now holding the stick in the same manner, gently twist your upper body sideways (16 times).

Keep the stick as in exercise 2, breathe out and try to bend forward till your navel line then breathe in and stand straight. Relax (8 times).

Stand across a wall and raise one of your feet ½" above the ground while breathing in. Breathe out and kick leg up till your hip line. Breathe in and bring the leg down. Repeat this with another leg (16 times each).

Lie down on your back keeping your hands behind your neck.

Take a deep breath. While breathing out, pull your left knee close to your chest and simultaneously twist it gently so that it touches your right elbow. Breathe in and relax. Repeat this for the right knee (20 times each).

Lie down on your stomach keeping your hands behind your neck and feet together. Breathe out and lift your upper body gently with chin up, elbows stretched behind and back arched. Breathe in and then come to the original position and relax (10 times).

Diet for the third week:
Repeat the diet scheduled for Phase I.

Phase IV (Fourth Week)

Do warm up exercises as in Phase III.

Spot walk slowly, arms rotating back and forth. Breathe in and breathe out (7-8 minutes).

Support lower lumbar region with palms, heels facing each other, breathe out, arch your back and stretch behind. Breathe in and return to the original position. Keeping your palms on your waist bend backwards and then stand straight (8 times).

Repeat the exercise 2, 3, and 4 of phase III.

Breathe in and stretch your body upwards. Breathe out and then bend downwards to touch your feet. Breathe in and half squat. Breathe out and stretch with head suspended down.

Start mock skipping for 2 minutes as it helps in blood circulation, stimulation and is good for the lymphatic system. Then spot walk for 1 minute, hands opening and closing horizontally and start skipping for 2½ minutes followed by spot walk and 1½ minutes with arms circling.

Do 2 minutes of slow jumping jacks. Breathe out when feet open up and hands go up. Then to slow down spot walk for 1½ minutes with your hands moving up and down.

Lie down on the floor and repeat exercise 5 of phase III and then lie on your stomach. Fold your legs at knees so that your heel touches your butt and then try to catch hold of your ankles thereby forming the shape of a bow. Take a deep breath and breathe out and move upwards. Relax (4 times).

Diet for fourth week:
Repeat the diet schedule for phase II.

Ten moves for developing a good posture:

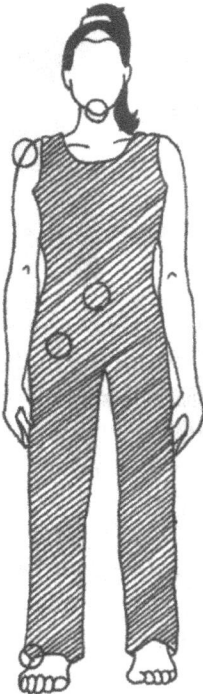

1) Stand straight with your chin upright. Make sure your shoulders are squared. Tighten your abdominal muscles and your pelvis a bit tilted downwards. Your feet should be flat and right under your hips. This is the foundation posture. Inhale through the nose and exhale through your mouth.

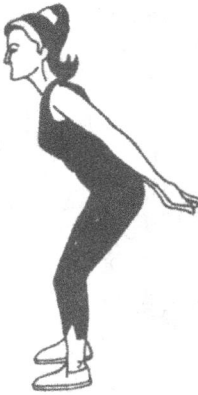

2) From the foundation posture bend slightly forward till you feel stress in your hamstrings and buttocks. Your head and neck should be in line with your spine, while your hands on your back. Pause for a few seconds, then squeeze your hamstrings and buttocks, as you stand upright. Repeat for 3 times.

3) Standing in foundation posture, press your big toes on the ground till you feel your thigh muscles contract. Focus on this muscle activation as you relax your toes. Now with your hands on your hips and knees bent, place your right heel in front of you. Squeezing your hamstrings and buttocks return to the standing position and repeat the exercise with your left foot 20 times for each foot.

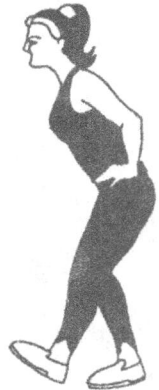

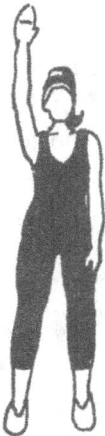

4) Stand straight and move your right arm in circular motion with fingers pointing to the ceiling, lift your right shoulder up squeezing your hamstrings and buttocks. Focus on using muscles of your shoulder and torso. As your shoulder completes the circle, drop your shoulders down. Concentrate on feeling the motion of your shoulder blade as you bring your arm and shoulder back to your side in neutral position. Repeat with other side too. 10 circles by each side.

5) Starting from the foundation posture, with your abs contracted, focus on the center of your stomach. Keeping your shoulders at ease and feet pointing forward move your hips in a slow circle around this center point: to the right, to the back, to the left and then forward. The key is to tighten your abs. Repeat this with other side too. 8 times for each side.

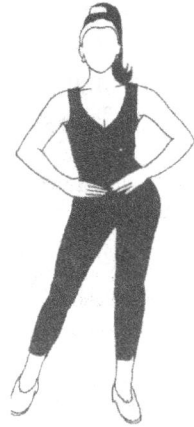

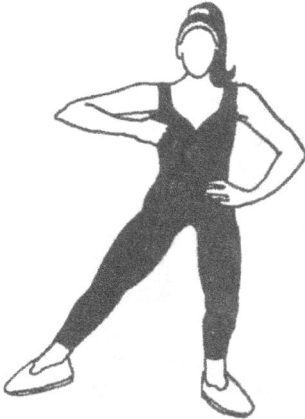

6) Stand straight keeping some distance between the feet, fold your right hand so that the elbow is in the line of the shoulder, close your fist and move it in the clockwise direction as if you're stirring a bowl full of soup. Repeat this with your left hand. 8 times with each hand.

7) Stand straight keeping some distance between the feet and hands on your hips. Activate your inner thigh muscles by pressing your big toes on the ground. Keeping your thigh muscles activated, slightly bend your right knee, with your shoulder, hips and knees pointing forward move your

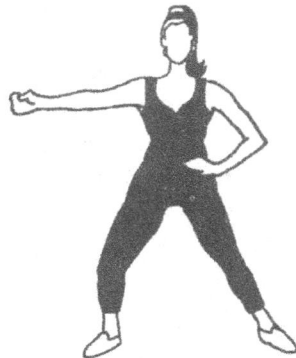

upper body to the right. Do not allow your hip to jot out. Squeeze your hamstrings and buttock to come back to the center position. Repeat this with left knee and moving to left side. Repeat 16 times for each side.

8) With both feet facing forward, combine moves six and seven so that as your upper body moves to the right, you bend your right knee and you make a soup-stirring circle with your right hand. Then change sides, so that as your upper body moves to the left you make a soup-stirring circle with your left hand. Use your hamstrings and buttock muscles for this exercise. Repeat 16 times for each side.

9) Standing in the foundation posture with your hands on your hips, your abs contracted and your left inner thigh muscle activated, bend your right knee, lifting your leg in front of you till your right knee is in level with your left knee. With your left hand press the inner side of your right thigh. Put your hands on your hips. Keeping your hips and shoulder straight while your right foot is resting gently on your left knee, squeeze the muscles of your left leg. Hold for a second and then relax. Repeat this with other side too 16 times for each side.

10) Standing in a foundation posture with your hands on your hips, raise your left knee so that your thigh is parallel to the ground and press your right hand on your left thigh. Move your left leg backwards and also move your left arm

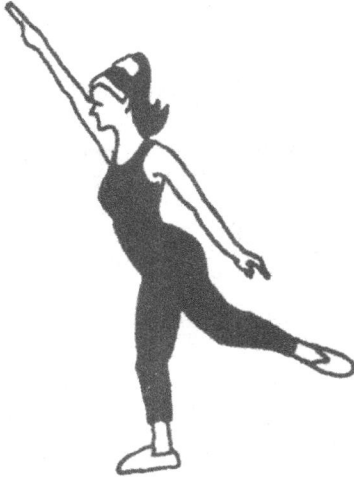

backwards and your right arm forward. Hold for a second, squeezing hamstrings and buttock bring your knee and arms back to the position with the left knee bend and the left thigh parallel to the ground. Hold for a second and repeat the exercise with right leg 16 times for each side.

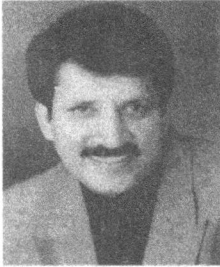

Dr. Sandesh Mayekar – Aesthetic and Cosmetic Dental Surgeon

Sandesh Mayekar is a known name. He is the dentist who helps you to put on a 'Million Dollar Smile.' While Sandesh is around one need not bother about one's teeth, be it the protruding and/ or a crumbling tooth. All you need to do is just give him a tinkle and get yourself that fantastic smile. He says, "What I work on is giving candidates the perfect smile—with teeth in proportion to the gums and lips.When a contestant is introduced to the audience, it is her face, her eyes and her smile, apart from her figure, that makes the difference. Now should the contestant have bad teeth she may not be able to give a broad, pleasant smile as she is not confident and there are fair chances that she may lose her points. Healthy teeth are significant for the 'Miss Beautiful Smile' contests."

Sandesh came into limelight in 1995, when Manpreet Brar was selected as Miss Universe, Runner-up 1. Says he, "She had all the winning qualities, except a flawed smile. She was tall, an intelligent girl, with a perfect figure. I worked on her with minor changes enhancing her smile that brightened her hopes for winning the coveted title. The confidence in her smile was clearly seen and it made her appear an altogether different person." Since then it's been a schedule that the winners of the Femina Miss India contest consult Sandesh.

Tips for maintaining oral hygiene (After taking treatment)

Do not chew or try to break hard food with your front teeth as it may damage your teeth. Eat food that contains fiber so that while chewing it helps in cleaning teeth and also avoid injury. Begin by eating food that is easy to chew. Always chew your food slowly and eat slowly taking small bites. Avoid smoking and/or drinking any such drinks that may cause staining of teeth. Stop smoking at least two-three days before the contest.

Clean your teeth twice a day with toothpaste to prevent plaque build up and bad breath. There are various cleansing agents like bleaching, whitening agents to clear the stains if any. This is done two days prior to the contest. If possible try dental flossing and clean off the food remnants, if any. Gargle properly after every meal.

General instructions:

Visit your dentist every six months for a check up. Even if you have some minor problems get the treatment done. Dental problems need to be taken seriously. One cannot take pills and go on. Also remove the plaque regularly else it becomes hard and forms tartar and calculus alongside the gums, which makes it difficult to clean up your teeth and as a result you may get gum problems. Use an interdental cleaner once in a day to clean your teeth as it also makes your teeth shine. Use a toothpaste that contains fluoride; make sure it is anti-bacterial. Fluoride strengthens the teeth and is very important for increasing the immunity. Check that the toothpaste is IDA approved as it acknowledges the credibility of the product. Also use a mouth rinse. In fact, everyone above the age of six should use a fluoride mouth rinse. Dental flossing is also important. It cleans the food that remains in between the teeth which cannot be removed by toothbrush. It is also safe, as it does not cause any damage to teeth and gums.

Clean your tongue properly with a tongue cleaner. Use toothbrush of a good quality fiber where the bristles are not too hard. Do not brush your teeth horizontally but move it slowly up and down with slight vibrations. Change your toothbrush every three months. But if it spoils early, change it immediately.

Fluoride is very essential for teeth as it makes teeth healthier and avoids tooth decay. Our body gets sufficient amount of it from drinking water.

Acidic substance like lemon juice, sweet lime juice, etc. though useful for the body, may cause damage to your teeth and so always drink juices with the help of a straw.

While eating acidic food elements take care that it does not come in direct contact of your teeth.

Our mouth has a natural fluid called saliva that is formed while we have our meal and it neutralises the acidic substances and cleans the food remnants that helps in keeping our mouth clean. And so it is advisable to avoid eating between lunch/dinner. Also avoid chocolates, toffees and peppermints as this increases chances of tooth decay. Also it has been scientifically proved that sugar-free chewing gum is good for teeth as it lessens acidic reactions.

Bad breath:

There are many reasons for bad breath like improper oral hygiene, gum disorders, chest disorders or stomach disorders. Improper hygiene may cause gingivitis (swollen gums) and suppuration with a pocket formation between the teeth and the gums. This results in a chronic puss discharge at the margin of the gums. This condition is known as pyorrhea and is the common cause for bad breath. Under such conditions, consult your dentist and get the treatment done. If needed the dentist will perform a surgery. Take proper care of your teeth. Use toothpaste containing fluoride and triclosis. Have a balanced diet and eat fibrous food as far as possible to keep yourself healthy. This will help you to keep your teeth healthy.

Smile designing:

What is smile designing?

Smile design is just about smiling in such a way that it enhances your beauty.

How is it done?

While designing a smile of a particular person the movement of the face line, eyes, nose, lips are considered and then the best possible smile is suggested. Also, as teeth are clearly visible while laughing, the defects are to be concealed. Then there are smile exercises and face-lifting exercises to be followed.

Smile exercises:

Smiling is not a random or an abrupt action but it involves a systematic movement, retraction and elevation of muscles and so the first exercise will consist of producing a voluntary smile that will bring into action the muscles involved in the movements of retraction and elevation of the oral structure that will be rapidly controlled.

This exercise will produce concentric, eccentric and isometric types of contraction. Gibson in his 'Smile Power Institute' has advocated it and within a few days, by practicing five times a day, complete control of different levels of smile can be achieved.

This exercise should be performed slowly by standing or sitting in front of the mirror. The impact of this therapy varies according to the age of the patient and the type of pathology developed.

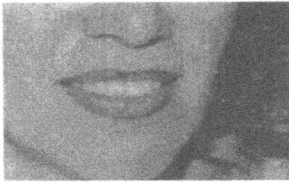

1) Have the face and lips in repose and the mind psychologically positive to slightly increase the contraction of the elevators.

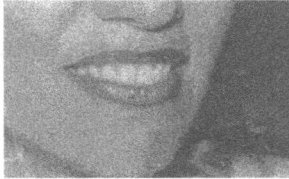

2) Begin to smile, stretch the corners of the mouth laterally keeping the lips in slight contact and maintain this position for 10 seconds.

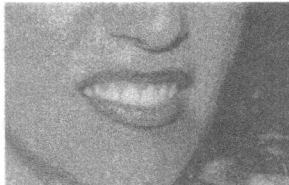

3) Expand the smile slightly laterally and upward to expose the edges of the teeth, control the parallelism of the corners of the mouth and maintain this position for 10 seconds.

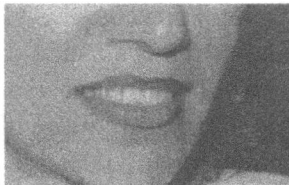

4) Increase the muscle tensicn, displaying a larger number and amount of teeth and exhibiting a lateral expansion of the cheeks, and observe that the relaxed lower part of the orbicularis oris follows the retraction and elevation of the corners of the mouth to cover the mandibular teeth. Keep this position for 10 seconds.

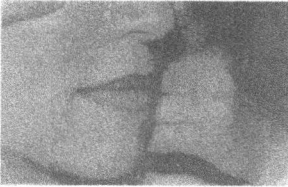

5) Give full tension to the muscles predominantly laterally, paying attention not to expose gingival tissue with the exception of the interdental papilla. Keep this position for 10 seconds.

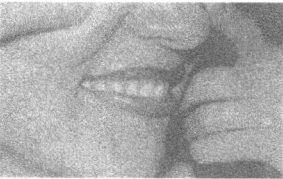

6) Slowly relax and maintain one half of the teeth visibility. Maintain this position for 10 seconds.

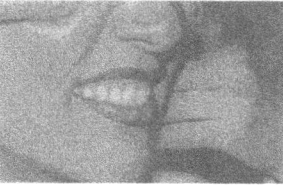

7) Continue relaxing, just keeping the edges of the maxillary anterior teeth visible and maintain for 10 seconds.

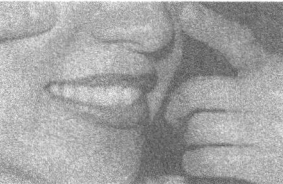

8) Go back to the initial position maintaining a slight tension of the elevators for 10 seconds. Relax.

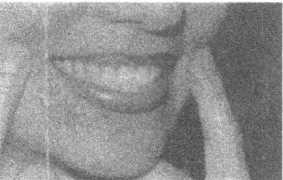

9) Form a full smile and maintain this smile with finger pressure at each corner.

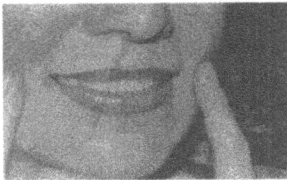

10) Close the smile halfway, with a finger resisting the pull and hold pressure for 10 seconds.

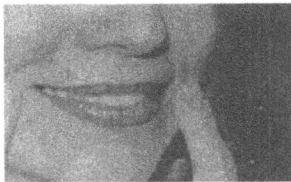

11) Try to close the smile completely with a finger resisting, having the lips trying to make contact in the middle part and maintain for 10 seconds. Relax.

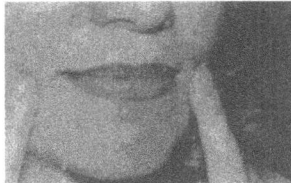

12) Reverse this exercise and place the fingers laterally at the corners of the mouth, slightly resisting muscle pull.

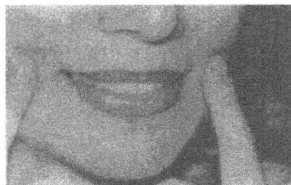

13) Maintain the pressure and try to expand the smile laterally and maintain for 10 seconds.

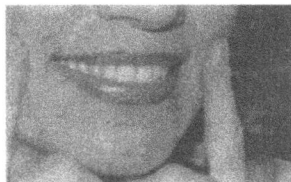

14) Expand the smile, reducing finger pressure.

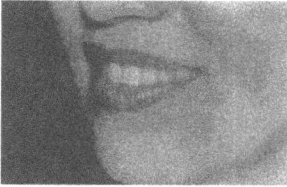

15) Relax and make a test.

Face-lifting exercises:

To maintain the muscle tone so that your facial appearance is not spoilt, it is advisable to perform face-lifting exercise after smile exercise, if possible every day.

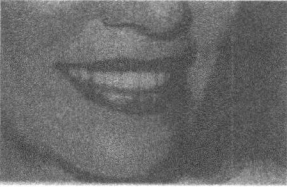

1) Have the mouth slightly open and flare the nostrils of the nose.

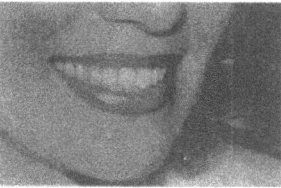

2) Wrinkle up the nose as far as possible and relax the upper lip.

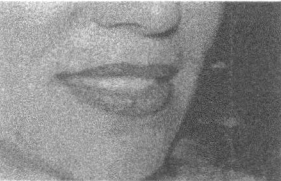

3) Slowly draw the upper lip upward as high as possible and maintain for 10 seconds.

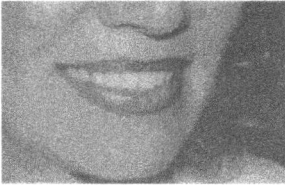

4) Concentrate on the upper lip and slowly bring it down. Relax.

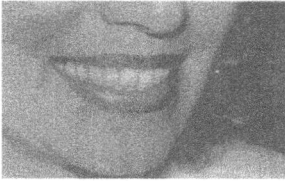

5) Have the mouth slightly open. Apply the middle, index or annular fingers under the eye on the cheekbone and relax the upper lip.

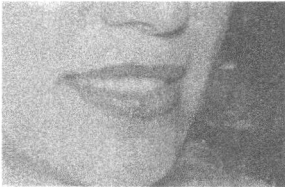

6) Curl the lip slowly up and maintain for 10 seconds.

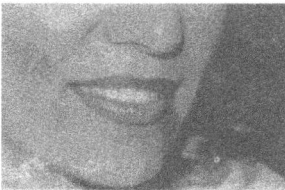

7) Curl the lip as high as possible, maintaining the finger pressure and keep this position for 10 seconds.

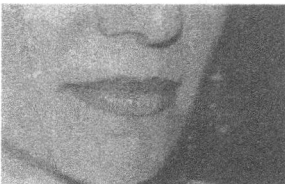

8) Return slowly to the initial position. Remove the fingers and relax.

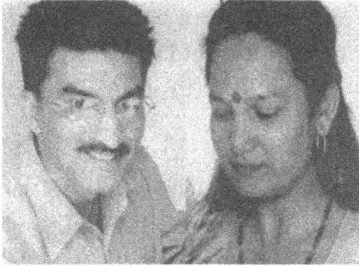

Bharat and Dorris Godambe – Beautician/ Hair Stylist

Bharat and Dorris Godambe, the hair stylist and make-up artist duo, with their experience of 28 and 15 years respectively, are associated with top models and film stars. They are an indispensable part of fashion dos and film glossies and have worked with almost every star of the tinsel town, from directors like Kamaal Amrohi, Raj Kapoor to Yash Chopra. They have also been associated with contests like Gladrags Man Hunt, Gladrags Super Model and many more. Bharat has done a course in make-up from London whereas for Dorris, it started out just as a hobby.

Bharat started his career as an assistant to Bollywood's well-known make-up artist Mr. Pandhari Juker, better known as Pandhari Dada, and was associated with him for 10 years. He was then a personal make-up artist of Parveen Babi. Things were working for him and then one fine day he met Dorris, they fell in love and married thereafter.

The duo, with lots of dreams to fulfill, started together initially with successful ad-campaigns like Lux beauty soap, Palmolive, Liril, Raymond's Suiting etc, and then on were involved with almost every big commercial.

They also worked on the official empanelment for the Femina Miss India contest. They worked on Sushmita Sen, Aishwarya Rai, Diana Hayden, and Yukta Mookhey, and to their credit all these beauty queens made them proud.

They both feel that over the years there have been many changes. Now, the look is more versatile. Earlier, one could see the use of just one or two shades but now there are over thousands of shades to choose from.

Says Dorris, "The right touch of make-up and hair styling can entirely change the way you look." Agrees Bharat, "Dressing up for an evening is not difficult. Irresistible party clothes complemented by simple make-up and hassle-free hair is all you need to create an evening look."

Bharat & Dorris' tips:

To create the finest look, imaginable for any occasion just follow these simple rules...

1) Wash your face either using a face-wash or by clean water. Dab your face with tissue paper. Cover your face with a little moisturiser and wait for it to dry. Apply the concealer to hide spots and dark circles. Put thin coats of concealer on the inner circle under the eyes, around the lips and other dark skin areas. The concealer should be one or two coats lighter than the foundation or else the face will look heavy. It should be applied only where it is needed.

2) Choose a foundation, preferably oil-free, to match your skin tone so that the skin appears smooth and flawless. Starting from the center of the face blend it carefully with a damp sponge all over the face especially the chin, around nostrils and under the jaw-line. Set it with translucent or compact powder for matte and refined finish.

3) Eye shadows accentuate eyes, making them look bigger and brighter. Use an eye shadow that compliments the color of your eyes. Apply the eye shadow right over the eyelid.

Draw a thin line of eyeliner on the upper eyelid, close to the lashes. Use a tipped eye pencil over the line for a smart effect. Apply mascara in an upward outward manner. To make the lashes thicker, powder them before the first coat of mascara dries. Then apply the second coat. For defined lashes use lash comb curler.

4) Even the prettiest of make-up remains unfinished without a blusher; it adds a little glow to the skin colour. Use powder or tinting powder. Dust the blusher on the apple of cheeks with a brush to give a natural look. Small brushes leave patches so blend it outwards with a big brush in semi-circular motions. Do not go close to the nose.

5) To give the lips a luscious look, first draw the outline with a lip pencil. Line them with a neutral colour. Blend inward to prevent the lipstick from bleeding. Use a lip brush to apply lipstick. Powder your lips after the first coat of lipstick. And, finally, use the lip gloss on the center of the lower lip to give the enhanced outlook.

6) Complete the make-up and then do the hairstyle. Hair should have a texture and should shine without stiffness for an easy and sexy style. Avoid using hair spray. For long and straight hair it is always advisable to leave them open. Wash your hair with a shampoo first and then use a good conditioner. Keep it for 10 minutes and then wash it with cold water. Avoid back combing for long hair. When hair is dry, brush it well in an outward direction using a soft brush.

Different hairstyles can be tried for short/mid length hair. For curly hair apply mousse while wet and crush it to create an instant hairstyle. Do not wash your hair on the same day if you want to style them.

For a sleeker look, toss your hair completely back and make a neat low bun or tie a topknot. To create side strings take a few hairs from each side, wet them and pin up. After 10 minutes remove the pins and let the strings loose. To make it last longer use a little hair spray. Add volume to your hair by using diffusers and drying systems that include dryers and rollers. Hair ornaments and accessories can be used to create a different look.

Makeover tips:

Always apply makeup in bright light.

Never forget to moisturise before make-up. Blend the moisturiser all over the face and neck. It helps to prepare the skin before applying the foundation.

Avoid using foundation if your skin is very oily.

Always use a clean puff every time you begin your make-up.

Use gel tint on the base skin to make the face glow.

For sparkling eyes, outline them with a soft white pencil.

For glittery outlook, apply silver or gold highlighter on cheeks, skin and eyelids.

Important tips:

Face: Depending upon the skin type either opt for 'Cleanup' or get the facial done once in a month. Steam is good for the face but should be avoided if one has pigmentations on face or dark circles around eyes. Soap is alkaline in nature, so use face-wash of a reputed company rather than soap.

Dirt easily sticks on oily skin. So individuals with oily skin should regularly wash their face either with face-wash or with water at least three to four times a day. While washing your face, wash it with hands moving upward (move your hands down to up).

If you have dry skin, then wash your face only when you return home. Do not wash face regularly. Do not use soap. Use moisturising lotion or cream. Depending upon the skin type, select suitable cosmetics. Individuals with dry skin or having a very busy schedule should get the facial done once in 20 days.

Pimples: To avoid pimples have a balanced diet consisting of leafy vegetables and fruits. Do not use oil-based or grease-based creams. Once in 20 days, get the 'Cleanup' done. Keep your stomach clean.

Dark circles around eyes: Try to sleep well at least for eight hours every night. If possible, try to sleep early. For dark circles around the eyes use an eye gel of a reputed company.

Palms and feet: Visit your beautician once a month for manicure and pedicure. In case you have a very busy schedule then manicure and pedicure should be done in every 20 days. In a cool and dry weather and in the winter season use a body lotion as many times as you want to maintain the complexion. To keep the skin glowing and healthy, body massage is needed at least twice a month.

Hair: Brush your hair from the scalp to the end of the hair, 100 times a day. Dorris bluntly puts it, "If you want healthy hair, chopping off the ends once a month is a must. Depending upon the type of your hair, use a suitable shampoo. While washing your hair, wash it properly so that shampoo does not remain in your hair, else it spoils your hair. Do not apply hair conditioner to the scalp. Apply it only on hair. Someone might have limp hair after using hair conditioner. Such people should get it done with hair serum, which is prepared in high grade beauty parlours. All jobs of colouring, streaking, perming or shaping must be done by professionals who understand and know the quality or feel of different kinds of hair. After such treatments, occasional oil massages, protein treatment conditioning and healthy food are needed to maintain glossy hair. Henna, for instance, dries the natural scalp oil, but gives an attractive auburn or gold-red sheen to the hair. It is imperative to oil hair so that this sheen does not come at the cost of dry and brittle hair. Instead of applying henna go for colour treatment. Massaging hair and scalp twice a week with aroma oil prevents dandruff and hair fall. Never pour oil on scalp. Oil should be applied to hair roots. One hour after massaging, wash hair, remove oil completely from hair and then go out for a walk.

Nails: Use a small nail cutter for your nails. Nail filer should not be hard and rough.

To remove cuticles, from the rough skin around the nail, it is advisable to massage it lightly with oil.

While using artificial cuticles, use only plastic cuticles and never use wooden cuticles.

Nail buffer should be at least 1.5 cm thick.

Always use natural hand creams. Use protein rich avocado or vegetable oils. Never use alcohol-based or perfume-based hand creams.

Make-up for Facial Types:

The oval facial type is generally accepted as the perfect face. The contours and proportions of the oval face form the basis of modifying all other facial types. Always apply make-up in bright light.

Makeup suggestions...

Rouge: Apply in a triangular fashion. Blend towards the temples.

Eyebrows: Keep natural.

Upper lip: Accentuate the natural bowline.

Lower lip: Slightly heavier than the upper lip..

For a long narrow face with hollow cheeks the aim is to shorten the length of the face and give the illusion of width.

A pear-shaped face has a narrow forehead, wide jaw line and chin. Here the aim is to create the illusion of width across the forehead and length in the face.

A square shaped face has a straight forehead hair line and square jaw line. Here, one needs to slenderise the appearance of the face and offset the features.

A heart-shaped face has a wide forehead and narrow chin line. Here the aim is to minimise the width across the forehead, and increase width across the jaw bone line.

A round-shaped face has a round hair line and round chin line. The aim is to slenderise the appearance of the face.

A diamond-shaped face means a narrow forehead, extreme cheek-bones and narrow chin.

The aim is to reduce the width across the cheekbone line.

Cosmetics used in facial make-up foundation or make-up base:

Probably no single item of make-up base is as important as the function of the make-up base. Its proper application creates a pleasing contour of face, provides a base for colour harmony, conceals blemishes and protects the skin from soil, wind and weather.

Skin tones determine the colour of the foundation base. Skin tones are generally classified as follows: Pink, olive, florid, cream, white and sallow.

Choice of foundation shade: In choosing the foundation shade usually a shade darker than the natural skin tone is desirable. For either a sallow or pale skin tone use a rosy foundation and powder to give it a glow. For a florid skin tone use a beige foundation and powder to soften the reddish tone. For all other skin tones (fair, medium or dark) select the depth of foundation and powder to blend with the lightness or darkness of the skin tone. Too light a foundation makes the face look pale and artificial. A little foundation goes a long way. Using too much foundation is undesirable as it gives a pasty skin appearance.

Selecting the right foundation: Foundation make-up tends to give a matte or non-oily finish. There are three types of foundation:

Cream foundation gives the most natural look and a longer lasting make-up. It is formulated for both dry and oily type skin.

Liquid foundation is a color suspended in an emulsion of delicate light oil. For quick and effective blending, apply it on one skin area at a time using long smooth strokes.

Cake foundation adds colour, a smooth and velvety look, and helps conceal minor skin discoloration. It is generally quite harmless. Cake foundation is applied with a moistened pad. It is very effective on oily skin.

Skin blemishes can be hidden with the aid of Stick foundation. Make-up in stick form is particularly useful in the covering or masking of minor skin blemishes. The advantage of a stick is that it can easily be applied to a small blemish and can give a relatively thick coverage. Blemish masking creams are similar to the pigment foundation creams.

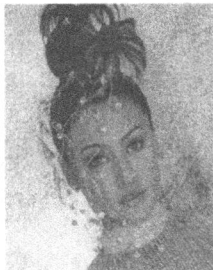

Namrata Shirodkar –
Miss India 1993, Miss
Universe-Runner up 3,
Miss Asia Pacific-Runner up 1

Now almost into retirement from active modelling, Namrata Shirodkar was one of the top choices in early 1990s. She was one of the models whom designers still miss and while on ramp, nobody could have missed her. Her presence was electrifying on ramp. In her active modelling days, she was in the top five models of her time.

Madhu Sapre and Namrata were school friends and it was on Madhu's insistence that Namrata decided to participate in the Femina Miss India contest. Her friends, Madhu and Mehr Jessia, helped her a lot. She was a beauty with brains. During the contest she was asked the final question "What's first, chicken or the egg?" She promptly replied "the chicken" and bagged the title Miss India 1993. Namrata became a household name then.

Daughter of the known model, Vinita Shirodkar, Namrata says, "It was more of my mom's dream than mine. She had done more than 200 assignments and just because she was married early she could not participate in the Femina Miss India contest. It was my family's desire to see me being crowned as Miss India."

Namrata's style at catwalk was graceful, simple and yet very glamorous. She was known to carry western as well as Indian dresses with elegance and ease. Namrata had to leave for the Miss Universe contest and had to prepare for it. Of course, her friends did advise her but there was something that was perturbing.

At the Miss Universe destination there were routine rehearsals, early mornings and late nights, nothing beyond practice. Namrata could not cope with the frazzling schedule. She was homesick, but knew that she was representing her country at the international level and could not give up and so she continued with the practice sessions.

Namrata was among the five finalists for Miss Universe and her question was, "What would you do if you happen to be immortal?" Baffled by the question she replied, "Nobody can be immortal." Very practical answer, but she missed the title and so she was declared as Runner up 3.

Interested in knowing Namrata's beauty secrets? Here they are:

Skin care: She maintains her healthy, soft and glowing skin under the guidance of dermatologist Dr Srilata Trasi.

Namrata's advice on maintaining face, hair, teeth, eyes...

Never wash your face using soap. But wash your face with water at least four to five times in a day. Remove your makeup with cleansing milk and baby oil of a reputed company. Use a soap as advised by your dermatologist.

Hair: Namrata washes her hair twice a week with shampoo and applies hair conditioner. For dandruff and any other hair problems she consults Dr Trasi. She uses the shampoo given by Dr Trasi.

Teeth and oral hygiene: She maintains it by cleaning it four times a day. She gargles her mouth properly after every meal and brushes her teeth every morning and every night. She had gums problem in her childhood but never after that. Namrata feels that it is best to consult a dentist for any such problems.

Eyes: She uses sunglasses while moving out in sun. Once a month she visits a beauty parlour. She gets the facial done, while doing the facial her eyes are covered with moist cloth dipped in rose water. She also does pedicure and manicure during that visit.

Diet: In the morning she has a cup of coffee and two biscuits.

She prefers to skip breakfast but goes in for lunch directly. In case she feels hungry she eats only fruits and coconut water.

Lunch starts with lots of salad, then two chapattis with vegetables and one bowl of rice. Sometime she has two slices of chicken/ fish. All these things are almost oil-free and a negligible amount of coconut in it. She never eats fried fish. Every day she drinks two glasses of coconut water after meals.

Four hours after lunch she has fruits and coconut water.

Dinner is the same as lunch. Namrata never eats potatoes or cheese. As a rule she has proteins everyday. She takes multi-vitamin tablets and B-complex tablets.

She maintains that it was just because of her mother's training that she could reach this platform. Her mother encouraged her to study dance since a very young age which improved her body structure and flexibility.

Namrata was always very good in spoken English and could boast of a sound vocabulary. She was well informed about the current happenings and had an impressive general knowledge. All this too helped her in increasing her self-confidence.

She acknowledges Gautam Rajadhyaksha's contribution to her career in modelling. He did her initial portfolio and did not charge a rupee for it.

Other contributors:

Beauty treatment - Dr. Shrilata Trasi

Dress Designer - Ashley Rebello

Hair Dresser - Madhuri Nakle

Photography - Suby Samuel

Namrata has a passion for designer outfits from London and the USA. Whether in the modelling world or in the tinsel town Namrata has been much admired for her hard work and dedication.

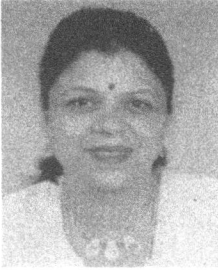

Dr. Shrilata Trasi – Dermatologist

Ever thought what could be the worst nightmare for a model/ contestant? Yes, the answer is getting a pimple on her face on the D-day. Why does it seem to happen when it is least expected? Says Dr. Shrilata, "It's just the tension and the stress that's creeping in, and also the effect of the make-up that increases the acne level, and as a result, a pimple pops up."

Her association with models over the years has been fantastic, but when it comes to her job it has been quite challenging. It's not that there are communication gaps but it's the short time period. Says she, "Technically, it takes three to four months for a standard acne to heal but that's a long period. My patients are demanding and I have to give them results in a stipulated time. They come to me saying 'Dr. I have a shoot next week and you have to make me presentable. Then I have no choice but to deliver my best and see to it that they have a clean and clear face within a week." Dr. Trasi also feels that a continuous exposure to flash lights and seasonal changes affects the complexion of the skin. To maintain the complexion always use a suitable sun-screen cream/lotion. Also one should avoid changing brands and should stick to a particular brand of make-up, of their choice, that suits their skin. She also warns against artificial hair curling/ perming/ straightening, for this disturbs the natural chemical composition of hair and thus leads to acute hair loss/fall.

Adds the doctor, "In their quest to have a beautiful body, often girls go on crash diets. Sudden loss of weight may lead to after effects like sagging of breast, rough skin or dull skin. It is always advisable to have a balanced diet and maintain our body. This keeps the skin healthy and glowing," she adds.

Dr. Trasi's tips on maintaining your skin texture at all times:

Flashlights, bright lights, sun, wind, rain, all these cause some damage to the skin. The skin damages are seen as you start getting sun allergy. It has varying clinical presentation. It varies from only redness to boils to sun induced acne, that is, pimples. Then sun itself causes rash on the sun-exposed parts of the body and if this damage is not taken care of, then one may get pigmentation. Removing this pigmentation is hell of a job. To avoid all this the girls need to use sunscreen regularly. Externally, there is no other way but to use good sunscreen with SPF that is Sun Protecting Factor. Internally, one could use antioxidants. Now antioxidants are the tablets containing vitamin-A, Beta-carotene, vitamin E and minerals like copper, zinc, manganese. They are now easily available in India. Beta-carotene has some sun screening effects and other components of this tablet make the skin rich in condition. So it is good to take them daily. Just one or two tablets a day go a long way. Vitamin C also helps maintain fairness and the texture of the skin. Fruit juices, salads, vegetables in one's diet help too.

Different remedies for different skin types:

Dry Skin: There can be many reasons for this and lets check them one by one.

Unsuitable cosmetics: Often when a cosmetic like a moisturiser or a foundation does not suit you, the earliest sign of a skin allergy could be a dry skin. Learn to listen to the language of your skin. Dryness is often the earliest sign of allergy.

Remedy: When you find your skin is drying, change the soap. If the dryness is not reduced in about eight days, then change your moisturiser. As a general rule, use cosmetics made by reputed manufacturers. Each cosmetic, however simple, has at least 40 ingredients, each of which has to be of top quality.

Heredity: Many people have dry skin since their childhood and this is a hereditary factor.

Remedy: Use a suitable moisturising soap or a body wash preferably, which is pH balanced. Use one that suits you and relieves your dryness. The effect of any moisturiser or cream will be doubled if used immediately after a hot water bath. Once/ twice in a week have a body massage using sunflower oil or olive oil.

Pollution and UV Rays: The UV rays are of high intensity and not only do they dry the skin but also lead to early and premature wrinkling of the skin.

Remedy: Use an effective sunscreen lotion or moisturiser. An effective sunscreen lotion must have a Sun Protection Factor (SPF) mentioned on it. Lotions which have SPF 30 or more are best suited for Indian conditions. There is a wide range of sunscreens available to suit every skin type, including oil-free gels.

Hard/rough soap: Generally soap by its definition has to be alkaline although the alkalinity may vary from soap to soap. The pH of the skin is acidic. Now if the soap is too alkaline it can dry the skin. Also the more perfumed the soap, the more it is likely to dry your skin.

Remedy: Use glycerine soap or even better a super-fatted soap that is neutral and mild. Supper fatted soaps have additional moisturising agents added to it that are not alkaline and thus do not dry the skin. For the face, it is advisable to use a suitable face wash that is generally neutral and very mild.

Some internal disorder, protein deficiency, reduced proportion of water intake, some hormonal problems like hypothyroidism, internal cancers like Lymphomas may be the causative factors for dry skin.

Dry skin problem is not as simple as it appears. Consult skin specialist if skin continues to remain dry for few weeks.

Oily Skin: Use a mild soap and a soap-free face wash. Try to keep the face clean by using a suitable cleanser followed by a face toner and astringent. Excess of steam bath may lead to Xeroderma that leads to dry and rough skin. During summer season wash your face with water at least three to four times a day.

Skin care (General):

Maintain good eating habits to keep the skin glowing. Avoid eating junk food. Be careful while choosing cosmetics and if you are the type who tries all the new cosmetics launched in the market, then you may as well say good-bye to your skin tone. You have to be careful while using face scrubs as they shouldn't be used on active pimples or the infection spreads. Scrubs remove the dead skin faster so they should be used in case of pimple scars and marks. That too they should be used sparingly, like once a day during summer and once in two days during winter.

Another thing that you can trust are natural face packs. Fruits and vegetables have natural Alpha Hydroxy Acids (AHA) that are good for skin. AHA has shown wonderful results on ageing skin, pigmentation, and environmental-induced changes like tans etc. Sour curd is another good ingredient for the face. It too has natural AHA and works wonders on face in few minutes of application.

Besan is yet another ingredient that is good for the skin. It can be mixed with curd or fruit or honey to show amazing results.

Remove blackheads and whiteheads regularly. Keeping the skin free of all these blemishes means taking care of blackheads and whiteheads. They are actually the early signs of acne. Our skin needs a constant supply of oil provided by oil glands situated at the root of the hair. As face is open it is easier for dirt to accumulate on the oil on the skin. This leads to the formation of blackhead or whitehead. As white head is a closed structure, it has to be cleaned. But a blackhead needs to be softened with the help of good steam to be removed. These days there are some specific creams that remove blackheads.

If you use a lot of bleach here is a tip for you—don't change your bleach constantly; stick to the one brand and use it once in a month. Bleach contains ammonia, hydrogen peroxide that induces pimples.

Pits are the after effects of acne. When acne heals what it leaves behind is a mark. So to prepare the body to face this damage we prepare it internally as well as externally by using sunscreen.

Pimples can be treated at any stage. Normally, there are three phases in pimple formation: a) comedons, blackhead and white-head formation, b) pustules and c) papules. As mentioned earlier, in the first stage having steam is a good option while in the second and third stage, one may need to take antibiotics and consult either a beautician or a physician.

Special seasonal care:

During summer, start with a sunscreen to prevent sun damage.

Take bath twice a day, as sweat and dirt on the body means that you start getting fungal infections.

Drink lots of water and fruit juices as we lose water by sweating. Also have coconut water, salads, and a light diet. Avoid papaya, if possible.

In winter palms, sole and skin in general dry out because cold takes water and oil from the skin. Most important things in winter are to use moisturising soap and reduce the use of soap.

Apply moisturiser after taking a bath to supplement the oil and water that you lose. Water is maintained after you have had a bath and moisturiser maintains oil. If this doesn't help then you may need creams containing urea like cotaryl or moisturisers or emollients.

For palms and soles you should keep a cream like emolene in your bag and apply it two to three times a day. If you want smooth palms and soles ideally you should keep them in hot water for 15 minutes to overhydrate your skin. Application of cream specially containing urea or glycerine, helps much more.

Massage your body with oil as it improves blood circulation, provides strength to the body and also gives a shine to the skin.

Dark circles:

Dark circles around the eyes are caused due to stress, working for long hours on computers, watching TV for a long time etc. Your eyes get strained, eye muscles get tired, blood supply to the muscles goes down and you get dark circles.

Inadequate sleep, hereditary factors (to give 100 per cent results is difficult here), malnutrition, inadequate diet also give dark circles. This can be seen when a person goes on a crash diet. So everything is finally co-related to the diet, mental state and your inherent body structure.

Dandruff:

Dandruff is caused due to excess oil that is applied to hair. When you have excess oil on the face it starts giving you pimples, same excess oil on the scalp dries up and forms dandruff. So pimple and dandruff are related.. The best way to keep clean is to use anti- dandruff shampoo once a week. The moment you find dandruff in your hair, start using shampoo twice a week and then on once in a week and later once in 10 days. However, overuse of anti-dandruff shampoo again leads to overdrying of skin, which means dandruff again. Overdry skin scales off.

Your face: Select suitable face wash depending upon your need as a number of them are available. If needed consult your physician/beautician.

Facials are advisable and should be done at least once in a fortnight. Avoid using creams with oil base as that would lead to pimples.

Manicure and Pedicure: Do it once in a month. Avoid overdoing as it causes infections of the nail root. Many a times girls tend to do it to suit their dress, which spoils the quality of nails.

Diet: Diet with vitamins, good quality proteins which you get from almonds, chicken (mutton should be avoided as it increases the cholesterol levels), eggs (give good quality protein but also increase cholesterol) should be taken regularly. Banana increases calories and body weight. Stick to fresh fruit juices and fresh fruits. As pointed out earlier, avoid papaya in summer.

Drinking water: Drinking excess water will be effective only if someone wants to reduce the weight. You have to keep your tummy full as alternative to food if you have three to four litres of water, which the dieticians advise.

Using soap: You can use a mild soap but more than that, it is better to use soap-free washes, which are available readily. Contestents of beauty pageants are young and have enough of skin oil. They should always do cleaning, toning because they are facing crowd, dust, dirt, pollution. For all these, three simple steps will help them out. They are cleanser, toner, and astringent application daily in the morning and in the evening steam bath or steam,once or maximum twice a week. It also causes heat-induced ageing of the skin so I would not advise it every day. Overuse of soaps will cause a drying effect of skin so it's best to use cleansing milk.

Make-up and precautions:

Make-up is a must for the beauty queen aspirants, but it's best to use a known brand and stick to it. Never use someone else's make-up which can lead to reactions and side-effects.

If pimples have left marks and scars, one has to get laser derm-abrasion by a plastic surgeon. Here we remove all the scars under supervision which we have done on one/two models. Yes, finally it is the face, which gives them every thing in life so we have to go to any extent to cure them. It is called face resurfacing which is done either by laser beams or by straight/brushing off so that the skin comes to normal. This is very effective. No body can ever guess that the model had a problem!

Miss Madhuri Nakle – Hair Stylist

"Hair is one of the factors that enhances one's beauty but if not arranged properly it might make you look awful. Hairstyle varies from face to face and many a times it can change your appearance and make you look a different individual altogether", says Madhuri Nakle. Madhuri has been in this profession for more than 15 years now and has helped many contestants look better. She adds, "It so happened that once Namrata Shirodkar was working for a photo shoot and I was just sitting across there. I noticed that Namrata was not comfortable, especially with her hair, and I just rearranged it for her. From then on I have always been with her".

Madhuri's simple tips:

Make a center parting followed by ear-to-ear parting. To tie a high ponytail do backcombing. For backcombing hold your hair straight and always brush in down to up direction. Now tie a high ponytail of the backcombed hair. With the help of bobpins and using a suitable hairspray roll the ponytail. Now take the remaining side hairs over this roll such that it covers the roll and then arrange them in a crisscross fashion overlapping on both sides. The center parting can be arranged in a zigzag fashion, or can be kept straight. Do the final touch ups using a hair spray.

This style can be used to look modern as well as to have a traditional look.

To have a western look put a tiara on your forehead while for a traditional Indian look have a tikka or put sindoor. To decorate put African lilies.

Hairstyle can change your look and make you look a different person altogether. It can create wonders and many a time makes you look incredibly beautiful. It can make you look emotional, serious, mature, lonely, mischievous etc. and of course can be used to show the way you are. It can be simple or very fine twined or loose or it can be melodramatic.

Hair Care: Use egg yolk, vinegar and curd in their original form on your hair as they act as revitalising agents. Also try to use leave-in conditioners (leave-in-conditioners need no washing, they evaporate within 48 hours) as they coat your hair and do not allow pollutants to settle on your hair. Also they maintain your hair tip and do not allow it to break open thereby always allowing you to take any chemical treatment and also ensure fine texture of your hair. Madhuri stresses on the importance of using Protein Packs. Pure Aloe, Redken, Zotos, Jolvel, Nexus are superior quality protein packs. They can give deep conditioning.

Crush and mix 8-10 dates with one egg and apply this mixture to hair. After 30 minutes wash your hair with suitable shampoo.

Wash your hair at least twice in a week and make sure your hair is trimmed once in six to eight weeks. Especially if you don't trim your hair when their tip breaks open then you have a fair chance of getting hair injuries.

Everyday we lose 50-100 hairs. As hair grow long their volume increases. Use of shikakai, reetha, mehendi gives glow to your hair but if you use them constantly over a period of time, they affect the texture of hair, making them dry. If at all you want to use mehendi, it's best to use leaves of mehendi, crushing them and mixing with curd and egg yolk rather than using the readymade powder.

Have a well-maintained and balanced diet so that your body gets the required vitamins and proteins. Zinc, iron, B-complex, potassium, magnesium are needed for body and they promote hair growth. If you lose too much hair then take one tablet of Sclerobion daily. Consult your doctor immediately. It is not advisable to have processed food and pure white sugar, as they are harmful to your hair.

To avoid dandruff apply a teaspoonful of oil on scalp and wash it off the next day. It is not advisable to tie your hair too tight as it breaks your hair. Brush your hair everyday slowly from top to bottom (at least 100 strokes). Use hairbrush with wide bristles to avoid injury to scalp and hair roots. Use castor oil for a change.

Once in a week get the deep conditioning done and wash your hair with suitable shampoo. Shampoo should be completely washed off from your hair. Before having bath tie your hair in warm towel. Keep it for some time and then wash your hair. If possible, avoid perming or applying artificial color to hair.

Remedies according to the types of hair:

Normal hair: Apply oil to the hair once a week, be olive or coconut or almond. This is called re-texturising treatment of hair. Keep the oil overnight and wash your hair the next day using normal shampoo. Apply conditioner.

Dry Hair: Massage your scalp with lukewarm oil at least twice a week. Keep it overnight and then wash your hair with mild shampoo. Apply hair conditioner. Once in a week do deep conditioning.

Chemically-treated hair: Such hair needs an oil massage once a week. Use a shampoo specially made for damaged hair. Apply conditioner to your hair with a special emphasis on roots and ends. Make sure you have applied leave-in conditioner before leaving your home. Once in three weeks take deep texturing protein treatment for your hair.

Oily scalp and dry hair: This is a very common problem and often occurs due to stress and dietary imbalances. Many a times it occurs due to overuse of medicines. Apply oil on ends without stimulating the scalp and wash your hair within half an hour.

Rough hair: Apply hair oil at least once a week and wash it off the next day with a shampoo. If possible opt for a protein treatment. Use leave-in conditioner. Go in for deep conditioning and protein treatment once in a week.

General tips:

For Indian women mid-length hair is the best option and it suits them well as they can get it styled with side partition or center partition. While getting a hair cut see that you have proper layering so that no matter the way you partition your hair, you always look attractive and presentable.

Do not use shampoo with conditioner. Conditioner and shampoo must be different. Many Indian women have thick hair. For thick hair protein treatment is a must.

While drying you hair do not hold the dryer close to the scalp or else you have chances of getting burnt. Hold it at least at the distance of one foot. Move the dryer in ascending order (from the bottom of the hair to the root). Dry hair tend to fly a lot so apply hairstyling spray or water on the brush and gently comb your hair. Before getting the style of your choice apply some water to make your hair wet. Use hair brush with wide bristles for wet hair. Wipe off your dryer with a soft piece of cloth. Do not wash it.

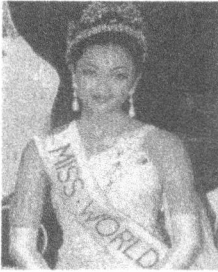

Aishwarya Rai – Miss India World 1994, Miss World 1994

She is the girl with aquamarine eyes and has made India proud time and again, be it fashion or the tinsel town. She has various accolades to her credit, like Miss World 1994, Most Photogenic Face, Miss India 1994, Screen Weekly 1997, Discovery of the year (Screen 1998) and Most Promising Newcomer.

Aishwarya, a serene pearl, shining in her own luster, luminous and aloof, holds her counsel as firmly as an oyster holds its treasure while shaping its destiny. Born as the second child of Vrinda and Krishnaraj Rai, Aishwarya had blue eyes like her grandmother and over the years they have turned to green-blue.

Being focused, she had an excellent academic record and was the head girl of her school and later on opted for a course in architecture.While studying, she happened to be in a shoot and could get into modelling without doing a regular portfolio.

But it was her Pepsi commercial with Aamir Khan "Hi... I am Sanju...." That brought her into the limelight.

In 1993, it was rumored that she had decided to enter the Miss India contest and certain section of media carried stories endorsing her as the face of '93. When Aishwarya did enter the contest in 1994 she made the headlines of almost every publication.

Aishwarya's close friend, Hemant Trivedi says, "Initially I did dissuade her. I think her entering into the contest was more of 'I want to feel good about myself' decision. Unfortunately, she was under tremendous pressure by trying to live up to other people's expectation and that's never fair".

Aishwarya has all those qualities needed to be an international model and she contested the 1994 Pageant. Every thing was going perfect and Aishwarya was doing a good job out there. She bagged titles like Miss Photogenic and, the coveted, Miss Perfect 10.

Then came the D-Day. Aishwarya recalls, "I can never forget this. I was forced to do my hairstyle on my own for the two rounds. It was only for the evening gown that I needed special attention for my hairdo and so sat down for it, as did other contestants. Time was running out and so unfinished, I just got up running on the stage, with my hair, the way it was. That was not the hairstyle I had thought of. I knew this, and even they knew it, as that was the incomplete hairdo."

As one of the five finalists, Aishwarya had the common question, "Which historical moment would you rewrite if given the chance to do so?" Quickly, Aishwarya replied "I would like to change the moment of my birth as, I could have been born with the qualities of the leaders of sort and would change the world to bring peace."

Her answer appeared self-centered and the pendulum swung away from her. The judges called for a tie and there was another tense round. But this time Sushmita Sen eventually piped Aishwarya by a whisker of just 0.02 marks. Aishwarya says, "In fact god was fair to both of us." But she admits that "When people expect too much from me something always goes wrong."

Aishwarya had to now prepare for Miss World '94. In the exotic and famed destination of Sun City, Africa, Aishwarya had to compete with 86 other participants. The day began and from the globe of beautiful women it was narrowed to the field of 10. The semifinals started with a swimsuit round and as Aishwarya came straight on to the stage, Richard Steintzman said, "Aishwarya Rai, Miss India, is careful about what she eats but that doesn't stop her from the occasional extravaganza."

Now Aishwarya was in her white gown, looking resplendent, standing on stage waiting for her question and had it. "What qualities should the Miss World 1994 embody?"

With the memories of her defeat in the Miss India Pageant, Aishwarya paused and replied, "The Miss worlds that we have had till date, have been proof enough that they must have compassion for the under privileged and not only for those having status and stature in the society. They can look beyond the barriers that men have set up for themselves—nationality and colour. We have to look beyond that. That would make a free person, a real person."

A spontaneous answer as good as it could be and Indians all over, waited with abated breath. The Second Runner up was announced, followed by the first, and just when it seemed like everything was over, Aishwarya could hear her name loud and clear.

Shock, disbelief, joy and finally euphoria showed on her face. It was certainly the most beautiful face in the world.

When Aishwarya returned in December '94 as the Miss World she received a royal treatment with thousands of Indians waiting at the airport. They lined the streets around her horse-driven caravan.

Aishwarya is naturally beautiful and hardly takes any special efforts for it. She takes care of herself, as any other regular person.

Teeth & oral hygiene: Uses a branded toothpaste and toothbrush and takes extra efforts to keep her oral cavity clean.

Hair: Uses products only of Clinic Plus/Pantene. Applies coconut oil on her hair twice a week and sometimes herbal oil. Also uses hair conditioner after having a hair wash.

Skin: Uses moisturising creams or lotions.

Eating habits: Eats oil-free food as far as possible.

Being associated with various charities across the globe she is also a favourite Indian star in Hollywood. She has terrific body language and she is grace personified while dancing. And yet this goddess of beauty still maintains, "I'm just an average woman with average concerns."

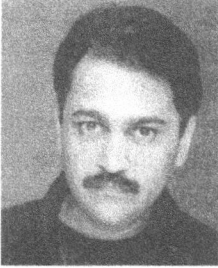

Ashley Rebello – Fashion/Costume Designer

Ashley Rebello is a costume designer par excellence. Starting his career as a manager with Benetton, Ashley moved to Bollywood with Mansoor Khan's 'Jo Jeeta Wohi Sikander', starring Aamir Khan. Ashley first made headlines when he did costumes for a Hollywood movie that was being shot in India. The star he draped was Hunter Tylo, most famous for her role as Dr Taylor Hayes in 'The Bold And The Beautiful.'

Ashley has worked with all the leading actresses from Juhi Chawla, Namrata Shirodkar, Aishwarya Rai, Sushmita Sen to Ameesha Patel. He says, "Every girl has her own style. The cuts and creases of garments you make for stars are altogether different than the ramp or catwalk. There is this absolute need to blend and gel designs to suit the character and the role of the star, or else it mars the entire character and presentation."

Speaking on Aishwarya Rai, Ashley admits that she's known to him since her modelling days. "We are good friends, Ash is a very reserved person. Being a model she knows how to carry herself. She prefers a very minimalist look, with minimum accessories," he says.

Ashley's tips:

How should a girl choose her dress?

One should wear a dress that suits her. You should just wear your attitude. It is not necessary that whatever is in vogue suits everybody. Most people try to ape whatever is in fashion, not knowing whether it suits them or not. Maybe flare pants suit only certain types of people but just because bell-bottoms are in fashion or Capri pants are in fashion, everybody wears Capri pants. If you think you look nice with straight pants or tight jeans or whatever you have been wearing and people appreciate it, stick to that and make your own fashion statement instead of aping trends.

There's no deciding body who determines what is 'in'? It just happens. I would not say that there is particular 'a' or 'b' person who decides fashion. To some extent, the film industry does set some trends in India, but even that is basically aped from the west or it is an amalgamation of the old.

Synthetic fabrics are a definite 'no' for Indians because our climate does not permit them. Travelling by local transport is not suitable for cottons because is does not look fresh. So preferably wear a blend—a blend that has more of a seepage effect, which will make you feel cooler. Go for comfort and go for fresher-looking fabrics that will not be creased and crumpled after travel. A lot of computer-based fabrics are coming up, where different types of fabrics are being blended. For instance, corn is being used as a fabric and it seems soft, non-creasy and really elegant. Soft textures are popular. There is also more awareness of natural-based fabrics like jute, cotton and silk.

As for colours, there is a lot of lilac, ice blue, and old rose, a lot of English colors. These colours were not heard of so much before, but they are all back into fashion. People are going in for more pastel shades and tones such as beige, browns, rust, creams, etc.

A working woman should have a black pair of trousers or a black skirt, a white shirt, a jacket in any muted, neutral color and a black top. If you have these in your basic wardrobe, you can team them with a lot of colours. For instance, you can team your trousers with a shirt and a scarf (that you can wear in the evening). Buy a lot of separates and team them together. It would be a good idea to own one basic black dress—it could be short or long—because black can be worn anywhere and everywhere.

A basic T-shirt and a pair of jeans, a pair of cotton shorts teamed with a little tying top and a shirt thrown on top is comfortable when you are relaxing.

There are a lot of boutiques offering teamed up salwar kameezes, where you can pick and choose the salwar or churidar, the kurta and the dupatta. This is really good because majority of the times you have these fixed sets, where you may not like a set in its entirety.

Churidars are trendier than salwars. If you have good legs, wear churidars, if you want to look taller, wear churidars; if you are stout, churidars will give you a slimmer look. On the other hand, if you want to look short, wear salwars, long kurtas. Cap sleeves are popular. They emphasise your arms, and so if you have nice arms, go for them.

Sarees in sheer materials such as chiffon, georgette with lycra, velvet or lace blouses have become popular now. Blouses can be in a variety of patterns, ranging from spaghetti straps to tie be-hinds and low backs. They make the saree sexier.

Plain sarees are more fashionable in general. Prints are going out; it is more plain or may be small print—like little motifs.

Footwear is strapping and open. For basic colours—don't go for colours that match the outfit. The size of heels keeps fluctuating. Right now, there is nothing as such that is in or out.

You can wear studs in your ears—may be a fake diamond or solitaire or pearl drops. It could be a plain chain, in silver or gold, with a little pendant like a pearl or diamond drop, around the neck. You need not have silver; oxidised will also do.

If it is more of a business occasion, go for simpler jewelry. If it is more of a social event, you could be more flamboyant.

Always remember "You should wear what suits you and what goes with you as an individual."

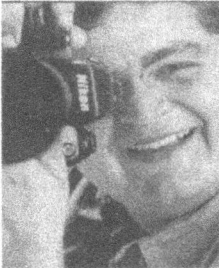

Daboo Ratnani –
Photographer

Daboo, as he is called, is one of the leading glamour photographers and has shot almost all the leading models and actresses.

Daboo has adjudged the Femina Miss Photogenic 1998, Hair Style and Body Beauty 1998. He says, "There is nothing like photogenic/non-photogenic face. It's all about communication. One should know how to communicate with the camera, especially in different angles/poses, express your feelings and definitely you'll have a good result. You have to be comfortable with yourself; your dress and you should be comfortable while facing the camera. It is not necessary that all those (boys/girls) with beautiful faces are always photogenic. Many a times I have done portfolios for models that are not conventionally beautiful/ good looking but they have exceptional camera sense and so they give the desired result." Daboo has shot many stars including Aishwarya Rai, Diana Hayden and Sushmita Sen.

Daboo's tips:

A model can look good by changing lenses, filters and shooting angles. One can make at least 40 per cent improvement but one cannot change 100 per cent.

Dress: Black, long fittings, vertical stripes can make you look slim. In case the model happens to be of wheatish complexion, avoid orange, green and yellow colours for they make her look dark. While colours like white or light shades make you look young. Dark shades make you look more mature.

Other tips:

Be happy and be in a pleasant mood on the day of the photo session.

Always have a positive and cooperative attitude, be it a competition or a photo shoot.

Put on a suitable dress and light makeup with hair styled suitably.

Be confident about yourself. While facing the camera express yourself clearly and try to communicate with the camera.

In case you are not confident, practice in front of the mirror for couple of days before the shoot. Do not be lethargic. Give your 100 per cent efforts and the photographer will give his 100 per cent and you get a 100 per cent result.

Diana Hayden –
Miss World 1997

Diana Hayden, the little princess from Secunderabad, bubbling with confidence and with her tomboyish approach made India proud by winning the Miss World title, for this was the fourth time in as many years that Femina Miss Indias have bagged the world's most coveted beauty titles.

Her parents did not try to stop her when she decided, at the age of 17, to leave her hometown Hyderabad with not a single rupee to her name. "I strongly felt," She recalls, "it was time for me to spread my wings." She touched base in Mumbai in 1992.

Diana sent her photographs for the Miss India 1997 and was the eldest contestant (23 years) in the pageant that year. During the 40 days training Hemant Trivedi taught ramp walk, Cori Walia taught make-up tips, Sabira Merchant taught the diction and voice modulations. Though Anjali Mukherjee was officially appointed by Femina it was Mickey Mehta who helped Diana and she could reduce eight kg. of her bodyweight in just 20 days.

Having won the 'Miss Beautiful Smile' in the earlier rounds Diana was full of confidence for the finals. It was clear from the outset that the contest was between Diana and Nafisa Joseph as they kept interchanging the top two positions in every round. There was a rare tie between them with 9.36 points each.

As rounds progressed the focus moved to intelligence and presence of mind. The question for the third round was "Why are women called the opposite sex?" This was again a tie.

Followed by this was a tie breaking question "Which historical figure would you like to marry and why?"

Nafisa won the round for her answer that she would like to marry Abraham Lincoln and learn leadership from him while Diana's answer was that she would marry the Late Indian Prime Minister Mr Rajiv Gandhi. This was the turning point as Abraham Lincoln was a worldwide-accepted historic leader.

Diana won the Miss India World title and was then sent to Seychelles for Miss World competition only to return as being crowned the world's most beautiful woman, at the Miss World pageant on November 22, 1997.

For the first time in the pageant's history, in 1997, all 86 contestants, instead of just the 10 semi-finalists, got the opportunity to appear before the panel of nine judges in their evening gowns.

Also the judges did away with the question and answer round, allowing each of the five finalists to introduce themselves in a line or two. Diana was easily the most collected of the lot, when she quoted W B Yeats "In dreams begin responsibilities..." and expressed the desire to help fulfill the dreams of others. She performed a hat trick at the pageant by also winning the Miss Photogenic title and the award for Best Beachwear.

Hemant Trivedi from the Sheetal Design Studio designed Diana's outfits for the event. Hemant, who also choreographed the Femina Miss India 1997 pageant, was chosen by Femina to groom Diana. He said, "Diana is very special for me and she has given me the best possible birthday gift ever. When she was first sent by Femina to me, she had what it took—height and great confidence, but was out of shape and somewhat podgy. We worked hard together and due to her perseverance, she started developing the required style and grace and a certain carriage and poise came through. We also got some dental work done for her. She knocked off a lot of weight in preparation for Miss World.

Confident Diana doesn't remember doubting her victory. "I knew I was good, so I never really thought about losing. And I knew that what finally mattered was my last answer—that was what would decide the ranking of the Miss World winners."

Diana has a distinctive personality. When asked about worldwide preferences of looks she says, "Grass is always green on the other side. While we love foreign looks, blue eyes, and silky blond hair they like Indian women, especially their black hair and skin colour."

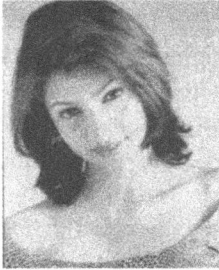

Yukta Mookhey –
Miss India World - 1999
Miss World - 1999

She is a typical Mumbai's girl next door who carried off the coveted Miss World title, beating 93 other contestants from around the world.

Yukta Mookhey, a 20-year-old zoology graduate, scooped the 60,000-pound top prize at a glittering ceremony at London's Olympia and did India proud once again, after Aishwarya Rai who was the honored winner of the tip title not long ago.

Graceful in her tight-fitting sky-blue sequined evening gown on the D-day, Yukta said she did her best and left the rest to God. Evening wear and swimsuits were paraded before a celebrity panel of eight judges, including world heavyweight boxing champion Lennox Lewis and Formula One racing driver Eddie Irvine, as competitors vied for the top slot.

Yukta was crowned by her predecessor, Linor Abargil, from Israel. Though she emerged a late favourite to win the crown, Miss UK Nicola Willoughby, 18, of Spalding, Lincolnshire, failed to make the final cut.

Yukta was appreciated all over, especially in hometown Mumbai. A six horse-drawn carriage took her to her home in the central suburbs of Mulund the day she landed in Mumbai as Miss World 1999. Prime Minister Atal Bihari Vajpayee congratulated her for doing India proud and the media lined up to talk to her.

Her family was extremely proud of her too. Says Mr Indralal Mookhey, Yukta's father, "Yukta has always been a disciplined girl right from her school days. Once she decided to do something, there was no stopping her. But she never disobeyed the family elders."

Yukta had some fine back up. She had her first portfolio done by Femina and Jatin Kampani happened to be the photographer. While M. Simp Roy was her dress designer for Miss India contest, for Miss World contest it was Hemant Trivedi of Sheetal Design Studio who designed her ice-blue evening gown, the collar of which was encrusted with Swarovski jewels. The Indian dress was made by Ritu Kumar.

Bharat and Dorris Godambe gave her tips on make-up and hairstyle. Theatre personality Sabira Merchant advised her on how to be witty, beautician Jamuna Pai on how to have the killer looks, trainer Mickey Mehta on how to have the perfect curves and Dr Sandesh Mayekar on how to smile with a sparkle.

While Michael Tung too showed her the art of make-up, Dr Rakesh Sinha, the gynaec-surgeon, motivated her and taught her to believe in oneself and decide one's own future.

The judges were clearly impressed by Miss India Yukta Mookhey when she said she would like to have been born as Hollywood film star Audrey Hepburn whom she admired for her "inner beauty, compassion and great aura." She expressed the desire to go to Paris, which she said was "so romantic."

Yukta's mom says, 'She had been dreaming of this since her childhood days but she took it seriously just before Miss India '99, that is, in September '98. The finals of Miss India was at the Pune Boat Club and the final question asked was "Had you been

Chelsea Clinton what would you suggest to your mom and dad that is, Hillary and Bill Clinton?"

Yukta readily answered, "Had I been Chelsea I would have suggested them to respect the family values and adhere to the family bond." Yukta was declared as Miss India World.

Ramma Bans, Mickey Mehta and Shyamak Davar helped her in maintaining her body and figure. Though Anjali Mukherjee was on-panel dietician, Yukta also followed Ramma Bans and Mickey Mehta's diet chart. One thing that she never missed in her meals was one spoonful of special chutney made of spinach, coriander leaves, curry leaves, salt, mint, garlic, lemon juice and green chilly. Also at dinner she had dal mixed with spinach.

Yukta's diet: Now let's check how she maintains herself and how she keeps herself presentable...

Morning: Glass of lukewarm water added with lemon juice and two dates.

Breakfast: Lots of whole fruits like apple, seasonal fruits like papaya, pineapple.

Lunch: One teaspoonful of special chutney made of spinach; coriander leaves, curry leaves, mint leaves, lemon juice, salt and chilly. A bowlful of salad, one roti stuffed with vegetables and curd (without cream), ½ bowl of sprouted legumes like rajma, gram etc. Everything, of course, oil-free. No potato and rice or bread at all.

Snacks: Fruits and biscuits given by Anjali Mukherjee.

Dinner: One teaspoonful of chutney, dal with spinach, one roti and vegetable.

Water: At least 7-8 glasses of water and lots of coconut water. She also has carrot and beetroot juice.

In case she feels anaemic she consumes iron tablets. She exercises regularly to keep herself fit. During the contest she used to have one multiple vitamin capsule and Becosule capsule.

Skin care: Yukta never uses soap but uses a mixture of curd, gram powder and lemon juice. In winter she uses moisturiser, hand and body lotion. She does manicure and pedicure once a month. She always removes her make up with cleansing milk and applies moisturiser. In case there are dark circles around her eyes she takes sufficient rest.

She keeps her face clean by regularly washing it and has proper diet and so she has never had any pimples. She takes due care of her neck and back. In fact her mom feels that it should be taught in childhood days to clean their neck and back, as most of them don't have the habit of cleaning their neck and back. This should be done by using a long bath brush or by using two separate napkins. Once your skin is clean then you don't have any skin problems like cracks or rough skin. Also Yukta takes due care of her feet as she takes of her face. In fact, her mom asked Yukta to start waxing her legs and get her eye brows done at 14. She says that it's a mother's duty to see that the daughter learns to take care of herself.

Dental care: She always brushes her teeth twice a day and cleans her mouth after every meal. She visits her dentist every six months.

Nails: She never uses any artificial nails but uses nail polish.

Hair: She uses hair oil sometimes and not regularly. She never applies mehendi. She washes her hair with a shampoo and uses a conditioner.

Yukta has been taking efforts in the right direction and is the outcome of proper upbringing and is still down to earth. While maintaining a proper balance she exercises for four hours in a day. She has been swimming since her childhood days.

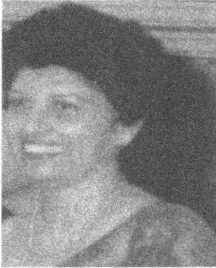

Aruna Mookhey – Yukta's Mother

Yukta has always accredited her success to her mom. Aruna Mookhey conducts workshops "Swiss Chalet" grooming for success and over 300 individuals have been benefited, including Yukta. Here the subjects that are taught are,

Motivation: How to set and achieve goals - success is a matter of choice.

Body language: posture, deportment, gestures (Non verbal communications)

Communication skills: Basics of public speaking and conversation, constructing speeches, vocabulary and diction.

Etiquette: Table manners, social conduct (Formal/informal)

Attitude: How to develop positive attitudes.

Interpersonal relationship: Improving relationships around us.

This involves lectures by experts of the likes of Sabira Merchant, Aruna Mookhey, Dr. Rakesh Sinha to name some. The workshop helps individuals gain self-confidence and develop higher self-esteem.

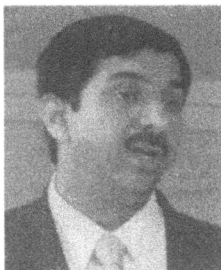

Dr. Rakesh Sinha – Surgeon and Motivator

Dr. Rakesh Sinha is the one who is known for his motivational speech and is the man behind Yukta Mookhey's success. He, who has been working on management and behavioural science over a decade says, "My life has changed a lot since I started implementing these principles, and I want to change the critical success factor."

Being a Certified licentiate of Neuro Linguistic Programming (NLP), he believes that verbal and nonverbal communication are the deciding factor for achieving success in one's life. Yukta was his first student. He feels that, it takes only one dream, one thought, perhaps an idea to change your life, and equally important is positive thinking. For success, one has to have a positive approach towards life."

He adds, "There has to be greater emphasis on various tools like strategy, obsession, passion, belief, persistence, integrity, values, ethics, communication skills, relationship and love. To achieve success in life, set various goals to be achieved. Success is all about motivating yourself to win and achieve everything that you desire in your life. Success does not happen overnight. It takes time and needs patience and guidance in right direction."

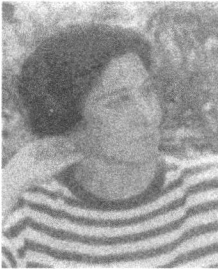

Ramma Bans –
Dietician, Beautician,
Fitness Guru

Ramma Bans is a health guru and beauty contestant trainer. With her columns being published in the leading publications, she is a known figure today. Starting in 1964 after her training in the UK, Ramma has been instrumental in revolutionising the concept of beauty in India and is still active at this age of 76, handling aerobics classes. In fact, she was the one who promoted beauty through health and has the credit of opening 10 health clubs over these years. Take a look at some of her spectacular achievements in the field of health, fitness and beauty:

1962: Started the first Health Club in India fully equipped with steam bath, sauna bath, fat-reducing electric gadgets, special facial beds and yogic meditation.

1964: Introduced herbal beauty ingredients in cosmetic preparation, oral pills for acne and pimples, tanning packs, gels etc.

1965: She introduced for the first time in India a calorie-chart, based on Indian foodstuffs listing their calories.

1968: She was the first to train deaf and dumb girls as beauticians thereby helping them to be economically independent.

1977-78: She introduced a health farm in India.

1978: She introduced the Whirlpool Massage in Delhi Health Club.

1979: She was the first to introduce aerobics, at the Taj Health Club, in India.

1983: She introduced meditation program and Shiatsu acupressure.

1984: She initiated promoting yoga through cassettes.

Ramma is also consultant to the celebrities like Sonia Gandhi, (even Late Mrs. Indira Gandhi) Rekha, Dimple Kapadia, Rani Jayraj, Linda Rana, Miss Universe Sushmita Sen, Miss World Yukta Mookhey and queens of many princely states.

"For a happy life," says Ramma, "one should develop a fit and healthy body, eat right, avoid stress, meditate to experience peace of mind and breathe correctly for life and vitality."

Ramma's tips:

Nutrition: "Beauty and health are directly related and much depends on your eating habits. Your diet should contain proteins, carbohydrates, vitamins, minerals and milk products. It should involve whole/skimmed milk, buttermilk and curd.

Meat, fish, lentils, pulses, eggs and cheese.

Whole wheat bread, chapattis.

Vegetables – Green/yellow.

Fresh fruits.

Ramma's height and weight chart:

A slim figure is desirable and pleasing too. And so it is advisable to keep a tab on our body weight.

Women		Men	
Height (in feet)	Weight (in Kgs)	Height (in feet)	Weight (in Kgs)
5 feet	46-51	5.2	56-61
5.1	48-53	5.3	57-62
5.2	50-55	5.4	59-64
5.3	52-57	5.5	61-66
5.4	54-59	5.6	63-68
5.5	56-61	5.7	65-70
5.6	58-63	5.8	67-72
5.7	60-65	5.9	69-74
5.8	62-67	5.10	71-76
5.9	63-68	5.11	73-78
5.10	64-69	6.0	75-80
5.11	66-81	6.1	77-82
6 feet	68-83	6.2	79-84
		6.3	81-86
		6.4	83-88
		6.5	85-90
		6.6	87-92
		6.7	89-94

Calorie control diet:

The calorie control diet comprises counting calories and rationing food from the approved list. This eating plan allows consuming around 800-1,200 calories a day and is approved medically. This also, in fact, allows to shed your weight by four kg/eight lbs in a month. While carrying out the weight control programs some dieticians suggest reduced water intake, which is not advisable. Even in case of dieting one should take care and consume adequate water, at least three pints, may be in form of water, liquid, fruit juice, milk and tea. Also one should avoid excess of salt intake as this bloats the tissue.

Slimming Menus:

Mentioned below is the chart for reducing the body weight and depending upon the weight you wish to lose you can choose a plan accordingly. This involves Indian and western food styles. Take care that you never reduce your food intake below 800 calories for more than 10 days, as this may prove injurious. The calorie contents are of approximate value.

Diet Maintenance chart for 1,200 calories - Non veg food

Schedule	Food Intake	Calories
Early in the morning	1 cup of tea/coffee with 3tsp milk.	20
Breakfast	1 boiled egg or a banana or a chickoo, followed by	80
	1 cup of milk/curd.	140
	1 slice of wheat bread with 1 tsp of butter.	115
Lunch	2 mutton chops or baked fish, 80 gms.	200
	1 bowl of salad with moong sprouts.	50
	1 bowl full of vegetable.	65
	1 fruit.	100
Evening Snack	Tea as stated above.	20
Dinner	1 leg chicken grilled or 2 pieces grilled fish.	150
	Boiled vegetables.	65
	1 bowl of salad.	35
	Khakra or 1 ½ slices of wheat bread.	90
	Fruit.	100

Hint: Try to avoid sugar and use Sweetex, if not possible, then use minimum sugar in tea or coffee.

Diet Maintenance chart for 1,200 calories - Veg food

Schedule	Food Intake	Calories
Breakfast	1 cup of milk with 4 tsp cornflakes followed by	200
	1 fruit, or 2 medium sized idli's and 1 bowl sambhar.	200
Lunch	2 chapattis or 1 ½ bowl full of rice.	200
	Dal 2 tsp.	100
	1 bowl of salad with moong sprouts.	50
	1 bowl full vegetable.	100
	½ cup of curd.	50
Evening Snack	1 cup of tea/coffee with 3tsp milk.	20
Dinner	2 chapattis or 1 ½ bowl full of rice.	200
	1/3rd cup of paneer with tomato and onion.	100
	1 bowl of salad.	35
	Fruit.	100

Maintenance chart for 800 diet calories: During this program you will have your food only once in a day i.e. either you have lunch or dinner only, and never both.

Diet Maintenance chart for 800 calories - Non-Veg

Schedule	Food Intake	Calories
Lunch/Dinner	1 cup of boiled fish or ¾ cup of chicken.	100
	1 cup of salad with moong sprouts.	50
	1 bowl of boiled vegetables.	65
	1 khakra.	90
	1 cup of curd or 1 cup of milk.	100

Diet Maintenance chart for 800 calories - Veg

Schedule	Food Intake	Calories
Lunch/Dinner	1 bowl of vegetable to be cooked with 1 tsp dal.	100
	1 cup of salad with moong sprouts.	50
	1 chappati.	100
	1 cup of curd or 1 cup of milk	100

Breakfast:

Mentioned below are the fruits in column 'A' and 'B'. You should make a pair and have it with tea i.e. to consume any fruits from 'A' and 'B' both. Be it in the afternoon if you are not having your lunch or at night if you are not having your dinner.

Column A		Column B	
Fruits	Calories	Fruits	Calories
1½ cup of Apples	100	3 cups of Watermelon	100
1½ Apricots	100	3 cups of Papaya	100
¾ Banana	100	1½ cups of Cherries	100
¾ Chickoo	100	1¼ cups of Raspberry	100
¾ Custard Apple	100	2 cups of Sweet Lime	100
6 medium-sized Figs	100	1½ cups of Strawberry	100
1½ cup of Guava	100	2 cups of Orange	100
¾ Mango	100	7 Plums	100
1½ Peaches	100		
¾ cup Grapes	100		
1½ Lichees	100		
Pineapple 3 slices	100		

On an average a typical Indian male (sedentary) needs 1,800 calories whereas a typically Indian women (sedentary) needs 1,200 calories a day. In case you exercise daily, then you can increase the calories (food intake). In case you need to reduce your body weight by four kg in a month then follow the diet maintenance chart for 800 calories. However, it is always advisable to consult your doctor/dietician before carrying out any diet maintenance programme.

Fibrous food (fibre) plays an important role in weight management. Sufficient high-fibre food in your diet will actually help your body to shed the surplus fats. But this doesn't mean that you can neglect calories. It has been proved worldover that individuals who consume high fibre have very rare chances of cancer and heart diseases as compared to the others.

Item	Qty	Fibre	Item	Qty	Fibre
Fruits			Food		
Fresh Figs	2½ oz	8	Whole wheat	1 oz	2.7
Strawberries	4 oz	3	White flour	1 oz	1.0
Oranges	6 oz	3	Corn flakes	1 oz	0.8
Plums	4 oz	2	Oatmeal	1 oz	2.0
Pears	5 oz	2	Peanuts	1 oz	2.2
Bananas	6 oz	3	White bread	2 slices	1.9
White grapes	4 oz	1	High bran bread	2 slices	1.9
Cherries	4 oz	2	Whole wheat bread	2 slices	6.0
Apple	5 oz	2	Baked beans in tomato sauce	8 oz	16.5
Prunes	1 oz	4	Spinach	4 oz	7.1
Apricots	1 oz	6	Peas	1 ½ oz	7.1
Dried figs	1 oz	5	Baked potato	7 oz	5.0
Raisins	1 oz	2	Lentils	1 ½ oz	5.0
Almonds	1 oz	4.1	Mashed potato	1 oz	4.7
			Cabbage	4 oz	2.8
			Onion boiled	4 oz	1.5
			Cauliflower	2 oz	1.4
			Chapati 1	1 oz	2.7
			Beetroot, boiled	2 oz	1.4
			Tomatoes	4 oz	1.7
			Carrots	4 oz	3.4

These are the only really dependable low calories choices:

Consomme—any flavour (lovely and clear so that you can actually see that they have not sneaked in extra calories.)

Oysters (for rich readers), half a grape fruit (for poor readers), A slice of melon any kind, any fresh fruit cocktail. Smoked salmon (if you can eat it 'neat' bread without butter) ham with melon.

Main course

Any plain grilled white fish (without butter), grilled liver, lobster, without sauce, plain grilled steak with salad, any seafood like crab, prawns etc. with salad. Omelettes without cheese, any vegetables can be ordered with these dishes, a baked potato.

Desserts

Ideally choose any fresh fruit-raspberries, strawberries, fresh figs, fresh fruit salad; everything has to be without cream. You can also have crème caramel without cream and ice cream only if it is simple. Do not have cheese.

Other tips:

To preserve the vitamin contents follow these simple steps:
Cook your food slowly.
Avoid frying.
Do not use soda while cooking.
Add limited amount of water while cooking your food.
Always cover the food while cooking.

Exercise

To keep fit and healthy it is advisable to exercise, if possible, daily. Always start with warm-ups like jogging, skipping, breathing etc. Various exercises are mentioned that will help you to keep fit and would also help to shape your body. Exercising increases body resistance and also make you look graceful. After completing your exercise do not jump to shower/bathtub immediately. Take some rest; let your body cool down and then have your shower.

Let's start with 'Surya Namaskar'

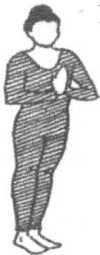

1) Stand straight keeping your feet together and hands joined at chest level in 'namaste'. Inhale and throw your arms back over your head and reach behind you. Push your hips forwards, keeping your feet parallel and toes pointed for wards.

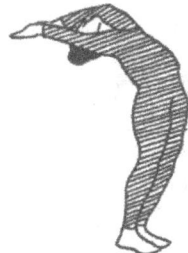

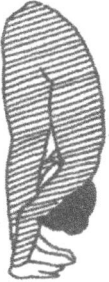

2) Keeping knees stgraight, bend forward so that hands touch the floor. Exhale. While bending try to touch your knees with your nose.

3) With hands rooted to the floor, inhale. Drop to your left knee, keeping right leg bent, knee jutting forward, and foot flat on the floor. Lift head, looking upwards. Let the right leg move backwards. Balance on your toes and Inhale.

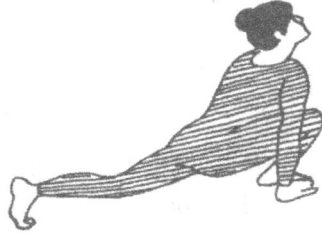

4) Holding breath, take the right leg back, and lift the left knee above the ground so that the body is in inclined plane. The arms remain rooted to the ground. Inhale and stretch out both legs behind you. Keeping elbows straight balance on your hands and feet.

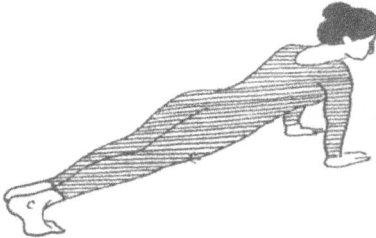

5) Bending hands at elbows, drop to the floor. The forehead, chest, knees, and toes should touch the ground but not the hips and abdomen. Exhale. The body is supported by hands, wrists and forearms.

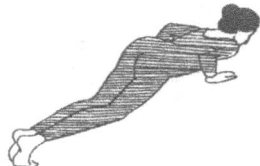

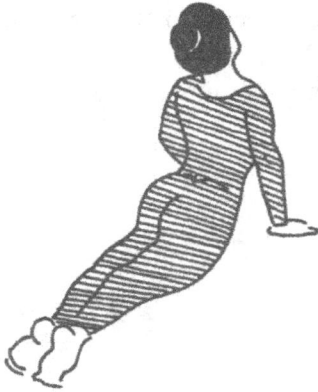

6) Straighten the arms; throw the chest out, curving your spine, turning your head up. Inhale and hold the position for the count of three.

7) Lower head and bend it down between arms while pushing hips up to form an inverted 'V'. Exhale while doing so. Keeping heels down on the floor feel the stretch.

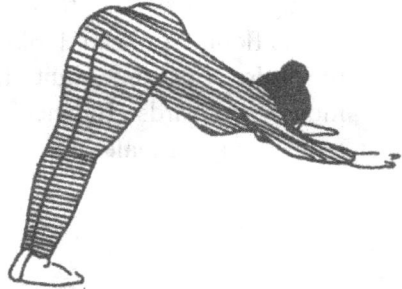

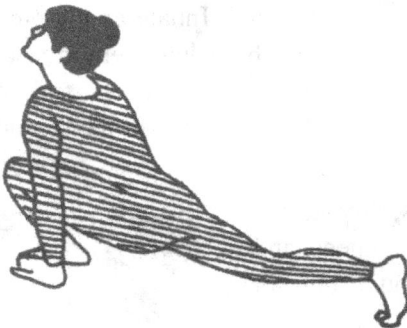

8) Straighten out, hands still rooted to the floor. Then bend lower, touching the right knee to the floor and moving the left leg forward, assuming the reverse position as (fig 3.) Chest out, look up and inhale deeply.

9) Move the right leg into position between hands. Exhale. Assume the same position as in (fig 2) by straightening both legs.

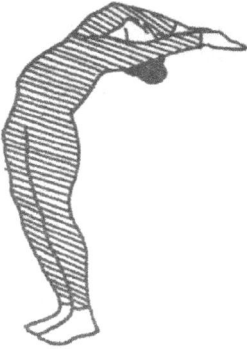

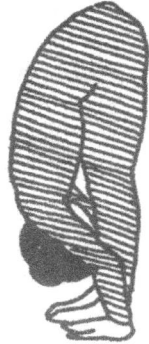

10) Straighten up slowly, inhaling as you do so. Assume starting position, Relax before repeating.

Start with three namskars gradually work up to 6. With daily practice you will find yourself going through the cycle automatically and as you gain suppleness you will also find that 15 namaskars are easy within five minutes.

The namaskar if correctly performed, will give you a glorious feeling of freedom and exhilaration. Do them every morning without fail and you will have plenty of pep for the rest of the day.

Now let's have a look at Yogasanas.

Trikonasan

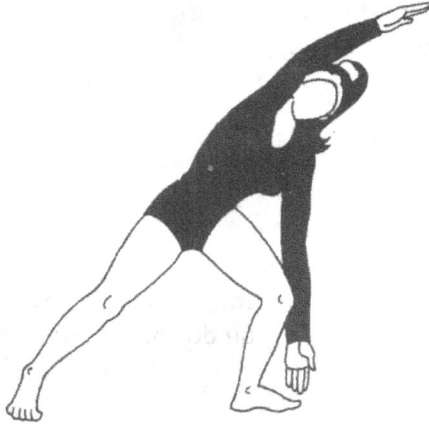

Bhujangasan

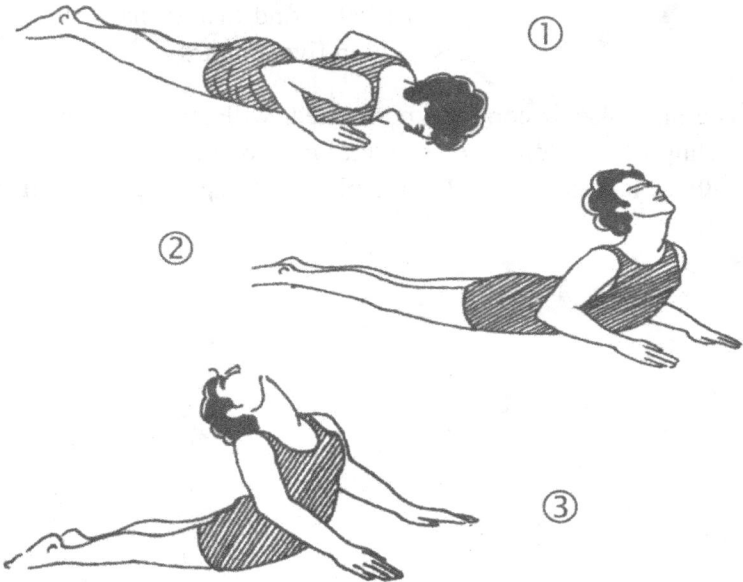

Paschimotanasan

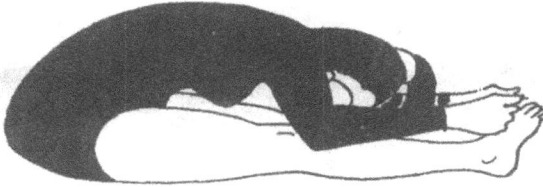

Gomukhasan

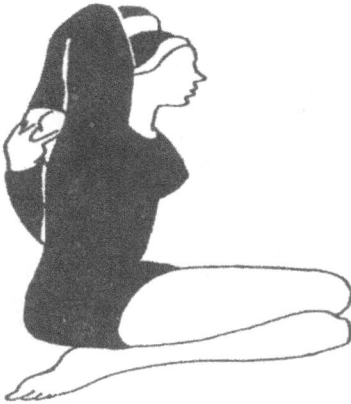

Veerbhadrasan

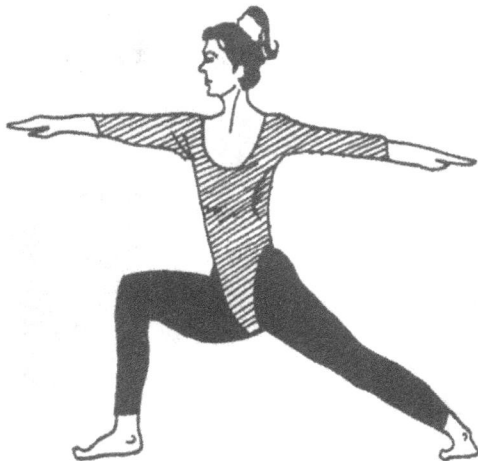

Upavistha Konasan

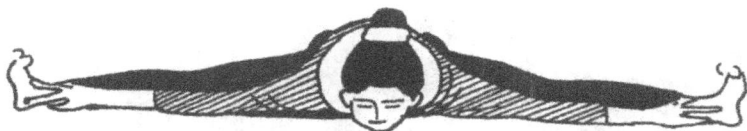

Halasan

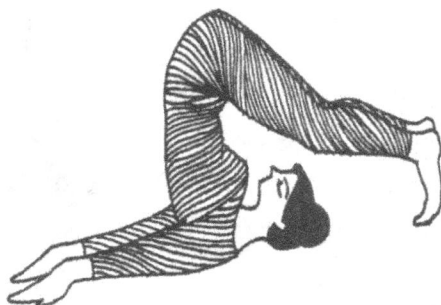

Tadasan

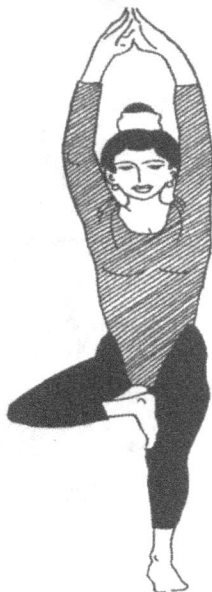

Shalabhasan

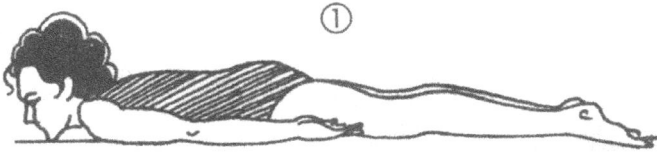

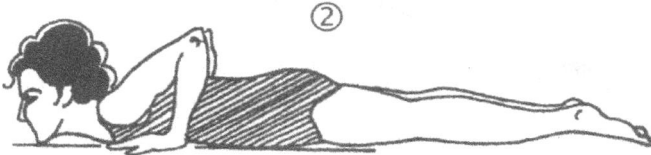

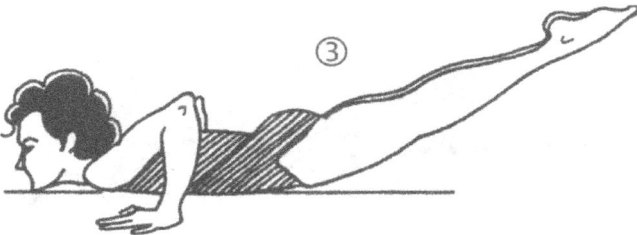

Pavanmuktasan

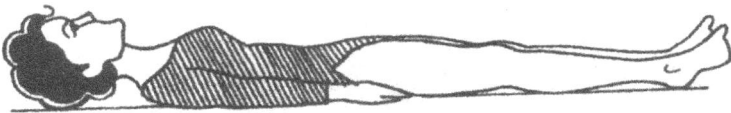

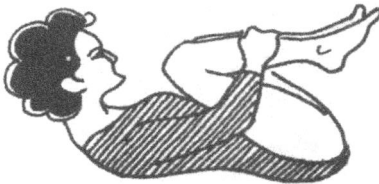

Naukasan

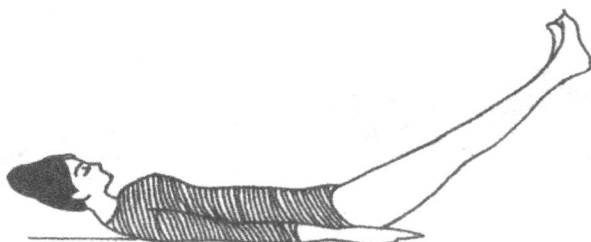

Dhanurasan

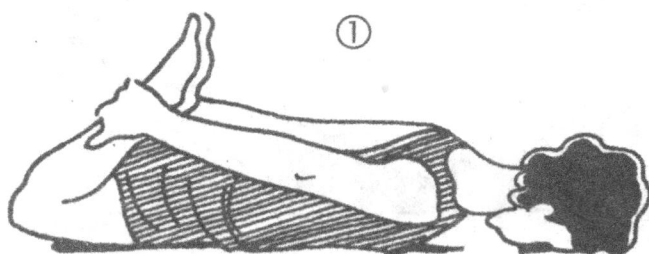

①

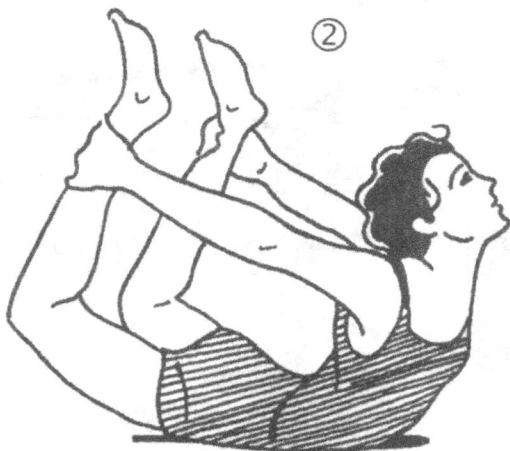

②

Urdhav Dhanurasan

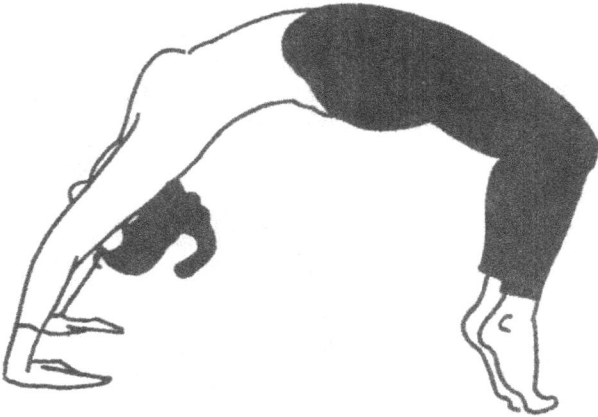

Janu Singhasan

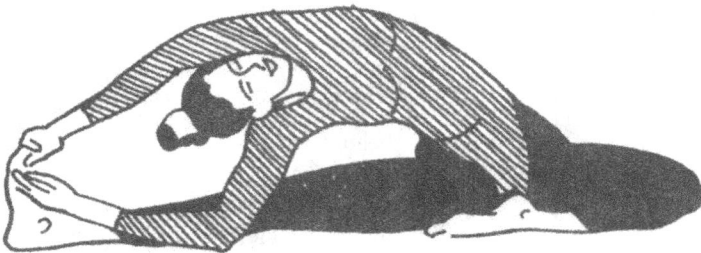

Part exercised	Position	Exercise	No. of times to be done
Waist (pose called The Triangle)	Upright	Stand with feet two feet apart, arms raised above head. Turn slowly to the left, taking firm hold of left knee with left hand and bringing down right arm, over bent head. Relax. Assume similar pose on right side. Go on to clutch mid calf and ankle after a few days' practice. Then do poses on each side in three consecutive smooth movements.	Hold each pose to count 15. Do the sequence 3 times.
Bust and back muscles. ('The Cobra') uplifts bust, strengthens back muscles, relieves tension.	Lying on the floor	Lie flat on your stomach with feet together. Place hands beneath shoulders, a few inches apart. Push hands and lift your body off the floor. Look upwards, keeping your hips just off the floor. Head back and curved spine.	Perform three times. Hold pose to count 15.
Shoulders ('The Posture Clasp') Improves posture.	Standing or sitting cross legged.	Bend left arm at elbow behind back. Bending right arm, raise elbow above shoulder so that fingers meet tips of left hand at back. Reverse positions.	Reverse positions 3 times. Hold pose to count 5.
Muscle of face, eyes, chin, neck. (The Lion).	Sitting	Sit on heels hands on thighs. Bending forward, stretch fingers of each hand taut. Stretch tongue out, opening eyes as wide as possible.	Repeat 3 times, holding pose to count 5.

Part exercised	Position	Exercise	No. of times to be done
Scalp. It leads to healthy hair.	Sit on heels.	Seize handfuls of hair by roots and tug locks backwards and forwards. Work overhead.	15 vigorous tugs.
Chin. It firms chin line.	Sit down.	Bend head back. Thrust jaw outwards and up.	Repeat 3 times.
Back, for flexibility	Sitting	Sit on floor, legs stretched together in front. Raising arms, bend to touch the mid calf. As you limber up try to touch ankles and soles of feet with hands.	Repeat 3 times each way.

A six-point exercise plan for individuals having heavy bottoms:

Part exercised	Position	Exercise	No. of times to be done
Abdomen knees and hips	Lying on the back	Stretch arms in 'T' position. Bend and bring knee towards chest. Reverse the position. Then bend both legs and bring both knees towards chest.	Repeat 8 to 10 times.
Abdomen knees and hips	Lying on the back	With arms in 'T' position, bend knee over from side to other thigh to touch floor. Keep shoulder flat. Repeat with other leg.	Do it 10 to 12 times.

Part exercised	Position	Exercise	No. of times to be done
Lower and upper hips	Lying on the back	Swing leg back and forth without bending knee. Then circle over-head with leg. Repeat process with other leg	8 to 12 times
Trunk	Stand, feet apart	Turn trunk round pelvis without moving hips.	Do 12 times each side.
Abdomen, thighs and trunk	Sit, legs stretched straight.	Lie down then sit up. Placing head on elbows, reach out to touch feet with both hands.	12 times.
Hips and thighs	Stand feet apart.	Bend touching both feet with hands.	12 times.

Consult a physician before starting your workout. In addition, to working the muscles aerobic exercise puts stress on the lungs, heart and circulatory system. Exerting yourself repeatedly and for short period at a time becomes conditioned and stronger. But for a person with heart problem it could aggravate the condition. To get the heart and muscles ready for action you have to raise your body temperature. The best way to do this is by gently stretching the muscles, warming them, thereby preventing muscle stiffness and injury. All yogic exercises are based on a formula of stretching, relaxation and deep breathing. Though aerobics taxes the heart and leg muscles it is important to do it too. Let's check it:

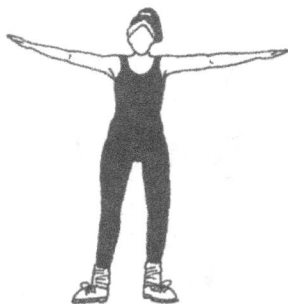

Arms: Extend your lower arm (through a downward arc) out to a shoulder height. Try not to move your shoulders

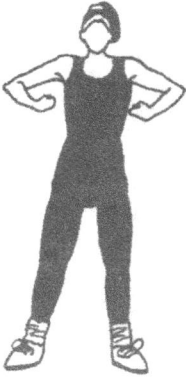

or upper arms and keep your palms facing the back wall.

Arms: Elbow extensions standing with knees straight; raise your elbows out to the side at shoulder height. Your lower arm is bent in towards your body; fists are clenched, palms facing the wall.

Waist: Sitting on the floor, open your legs as wide as you can. Point your toes. Pull over the right side—with both arms extending towards right. Repeat towards left.

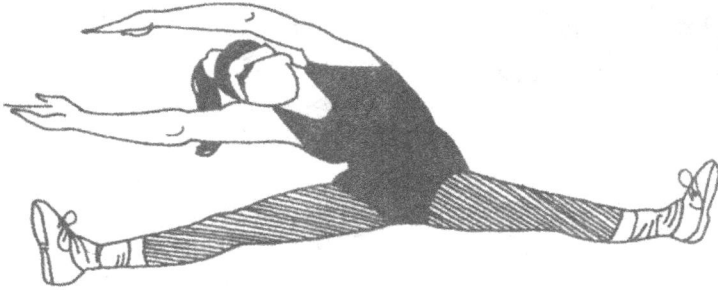

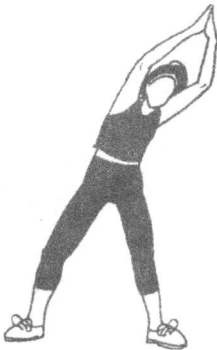

Waist: Stand with your legs two feet apart, toes pointing on the side. Stretch, hold hands and bend on left count of two and right count of two. Repeat 12 times.

Waist: Standing with knees straight, legs together, raise your arms to shoulder height. Hold hand in front, palms facing down, bending your elbows. Bend your leg, bringing knee to elbow. Repeat alternate legs 12 times.

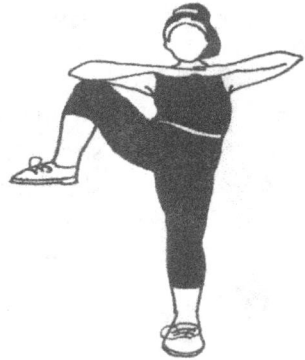

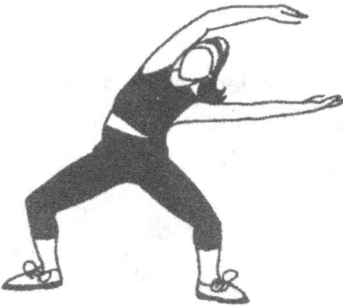

Waist: Stand as shown in fig., that is, 90 into deep PLIE-left arm straight to shoulder level, right arm over your head, bend waist and stretch left with both arms, Repeat other side. Alternate 12 times.

Waist: 90 into deep PLIE - right hand on abdomen, left hand over your head, stretch to right, bending your waist. Alternate 12 times.

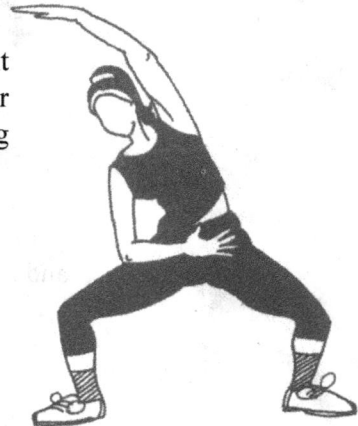

Waist: 90 into deep PLIE, right elbow on right knee. Left arm straight, look at your left hand. Repeat other side. Alternate 12 times.

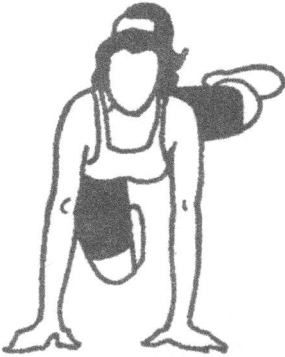

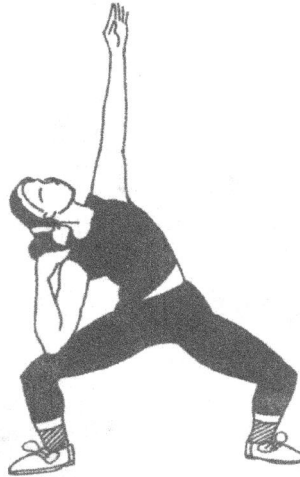

Hips and legs: On your hands and knees, weight evenly distributed, back flat, stomach pulled in, head up. Lift your right knee out to the side, bend and raise it to the hip level, thigh parallel to the floor. Lower your right knee down again but don't touch the floor. Repeat 12 times each leg.

Hips and legs: With left leg and right hand on floor pointing opposite, bend right leg, heel touching the hip, extending left arm hold right foot. Count 12 and repeat other side.

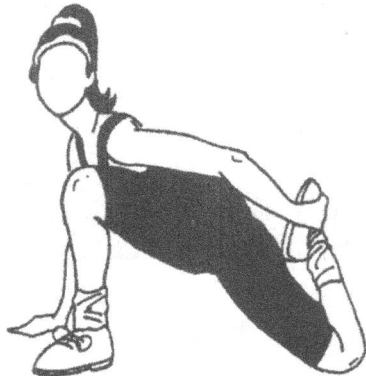

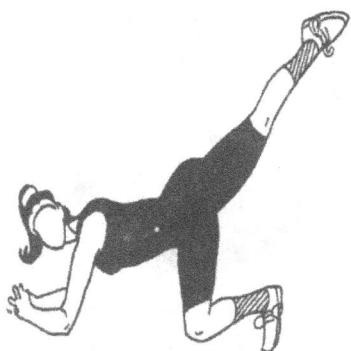

Hips and legs: Extend the right leg straight behind with your toes pointed and lift it as high as you can, releasing it slightly. Do it 12 times and repeat with other leg.

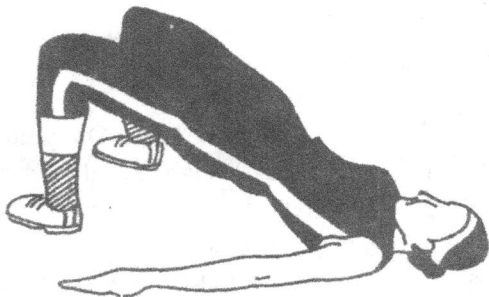

Hips: Lie on your back with feet parallel a little more than hip distance, stretch your arms lying alongside, shift your weight onto your shoulders and lift your buttock up. Do not squeeze and release your buttocks in a lifted position. Repeat it 12 times.

Inner thighs: Bend your knees into a squatting position and place your hands behind your feet. Your inner knees should rest on your elbows. Take small bounces with your buttocks for 16 counts.

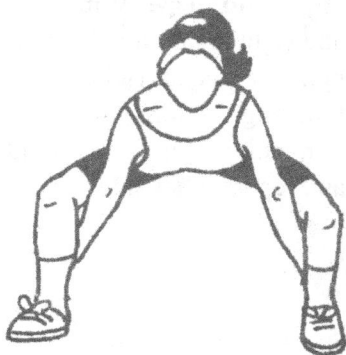

Inner thighs: Lie down on your back as shown in the fig, lifting your head up, raise your legs and stretch them wide open. Count for 16 times and relax.

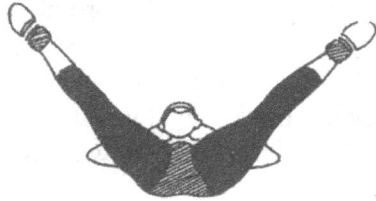

Thighs: Bend your right leg to right angle with toe pointing opposite - left leg stretch on your heels hands in front. Bounce 16 times. Repeat other side.

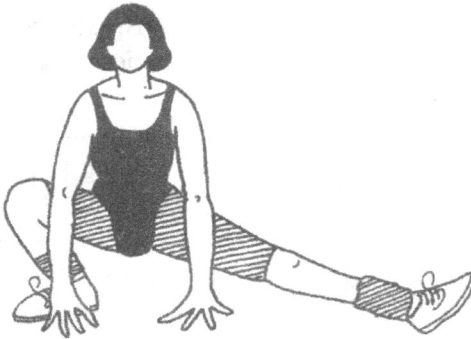

Abdomen: Lie down on your back; straighten both legs, perpendicular cross legs. Try to reach right elbow to left knee and left to right. Repeat 12 times.

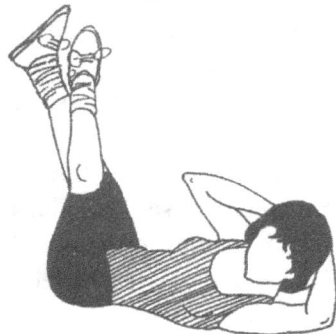

The Classic Six Western style:

Waist trimmer: Stand with legs apart, hands together at the back of neck, elbows down. Without moving hips, twist the top part of the body as far to the left as you can go. Go back to the original pose and move as far back to the right as you can. Repeat 10 to 20 times.

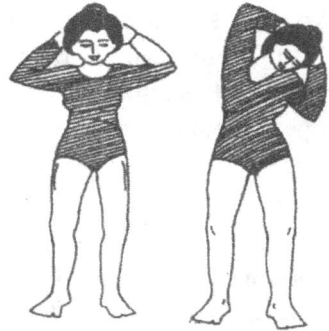

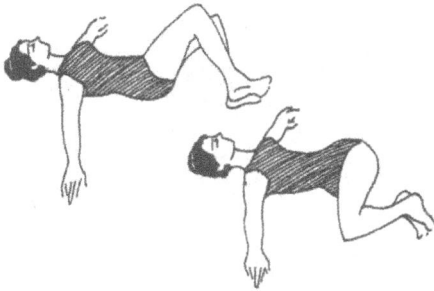

Hip swing: Lie on back, knees bent and raised slightly off the floor, arms out in 'T' position. Swing knees from left to right, rolling over so that the thighs come down hard on the floor. Start with eight swings on each side and work up to 15.

Tummy tightener: Lie on a floor. Raise your-self to a sitting position without touching arms, elbows, or hands to the floor. Repeat 10 times. Now lie flat as directed. Raise both legs at right angles to the body. Then slowly lower the feet. Do this 10 times.

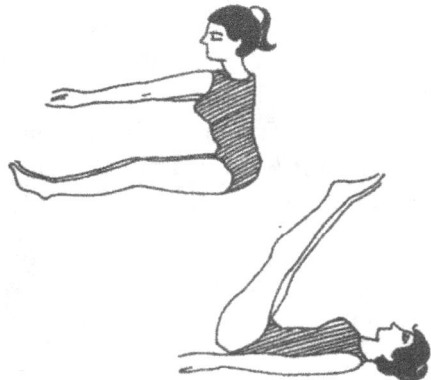

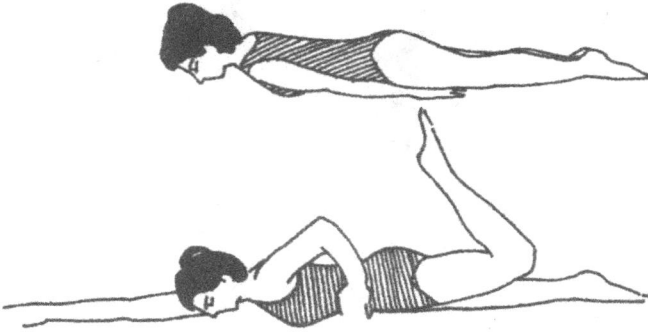

Bust firmer: Lie across the bed, face down, and see that you are suspended from the waist for your breast. Crawl and proceed with the over land stroke. Pull one elbow out slowly, reach forward, fingers together, and pull back hard. Roll and begin the other arm stroke. Keep a flow of motion. Count 100 strokes breathing in at every two strokes and exhaling on the next two. This is like swimming on bed.

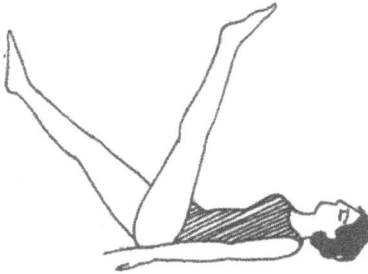

Thigh control: Lie on the floor, arms out at sides, legs at right angles to the body, spread legs wide, bring together. Do this nonstop 20 times.

Bottom level: Kneel with hands overhead, fingers touching. Keep body facing forward. Lower buttocks to touch floor on right, then swing to left and down. Do this 5 times each way working up to 10.

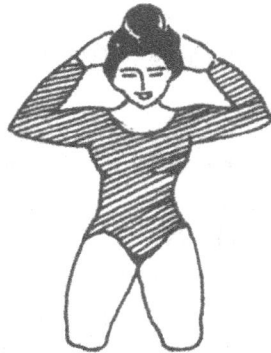

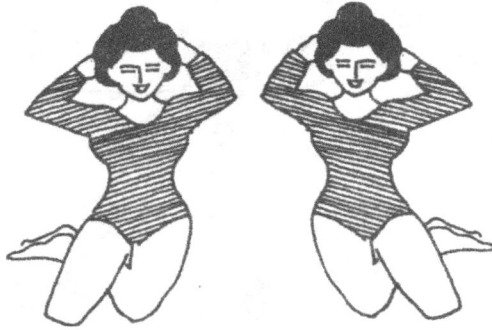

Last resort: If you cannot find time for many yogic exercises, do at least these limbering asanas, which my yogic students perform as a warm-up before their routine. Rotate the left and then the right shoulder in a clockwise and then in an anti-clockwise direction with the arms bent at elbows, fingertips touching the shoulders, three times each way. Then rotate both shoulders simultaneously, hunching the shoulders at the back while you exercise. Repeat three times.

Raise arms, and in a loose rolling motion, swing them upward, side ways, down, forward almost touching the floor. Then work sideways and back in a loose flowing motion. Now stretch your arms above the head and fall limply forwards at the waist. The entire motion loosens the limbs so that there is no rigidity anywhere.

Natural cosmetic aids:

Here is a choice of natural home-made cosmetics. Home-made preparations, of course, contain no preservatives. They must be refrigerated; even so they seldom last for more than a week. It is advisable, therefore, to make these in small quantities and to bottle them in screw-top jars. The use of china or stainless steel containers ensures that there are no damaging effects on the skin through chemical reactions.

Skin care

Cleansing agents: Almond oil is a fine cleanser. It is especially effective in protecting the delicate skin under the eyes.

For normal and greasy skin: Take a cupful of curd, one teaspoon of orange juice and one tea spoon of lemon juice and mix well together. Apply with fingertips and then wipe it with damp tissue. Splash skin with cold water and dry gently. A cleanser, which whitens the skin, is a mixture of the juice of one lemon with equal parts of milk and cucumber juice.

For dry skin: Make a cleanser of cooked oatmeal mixed with honey. Rinse off with warm water. A heavier cleansing cream comprises of four tsp of green olive oil, two tsp til oil (seasame oil), two tsp lard or any vegetable fat, mixed with two drops of any essence. Crush the ingredients till creamy. Refrigerate.

Face fresheners and astringents: To tone the skin, take half a slice of cucumber. Apply it over the face in firm circular motions. Allow it to dry naturally and then wash it.

Add one tsp of peppermint or pudina leaves to a cup of boiling water. Keep for half an hour, strain and bottle it when cool. Use after cleansing. A few drops of spirit of camphor added to the last rinsing water also acts as an astringent. Any chemist can make it for you: one tsp spirit of camphor, two and a half ounce fluid witch hazel, two and a half ounce orange flower water and two and a half ounce distilled water. Shake well before use.

Moisturisers: Wash eight lettuce leaves and boil it in a pint of water. Cool and strain through muslin. Bottle it. Apply with cotton wool pads dipped in a solution using light upward movements. Leave on for three minutes before tissuing off. Mix equal parts of rose water, glycerine and lemon juice. Take an ounce of almonds or cashew nuts. Dip them alternately in boiling water and cold water to peel. Grind to a paste. Add half a pint of distilled water, drop by drop, till the concoction is milky.

Conditioners: Take one tsp of honey and two tsp of light milk cream. Beat till creamy. Leave on the face for 20 minutes and then wash it off.

Honey and almond cream conditioner: Take four ounce honey, eight ounce hydrous lanolin, and one and a half cup almond oil. In a double boiler, warm the honey, blend in lanolin and, as it melts, add almond oil. Stir well and beat till creamy. Leave a little on face and neck overnight.

To peel off dead and rough skin: Rub a slice of papaya or tomato into the skin. Wipe off with a rough terry cloth towel. Smear palms with cold cream and fine table salt and rub it over the trouble spots.

To refine pores: Mix one tsp of tomato juice with a few drops of lemon juice and massage it over the skin.

Sun protection lotion: Extract juice from peeled cucumber. Mix it with half a teaspoon of glycerine and the same amount of rose water. Refrigerate.

For blemished skin: Rub a raw potato slice on the skin. An effective anti-acne lotion is the juice of mint leaves applied on the skin and left overnight. Wash it off with tepid water, the next morning.

A basic pimple cream: Mix one tsp castor oil, one tsp glycerine and one tsp lanolin. Place bowl with ingredients in simmering water till well mixed. Cool and bottle it.

Facial Masks: The traditional egg mask is the egg white, beaten stiff with the optional addition of one tsp of honey. Leave it on face for 15 minutes and wash it with warm water followed by cold splashes.

Half a tsp of lemon juice added to egg white benefits greasy skin. A whisked yolk of egg with a few drops of vegetable oil and a squeeze of lemon juice is fine for dry skin. A tablespoon of skimmed milk added to egg nourishes the skin.

Another great restorer is the honey mask. Take one tsp of honey, the yolk of one egg and one tsp of olive oil. Beat the yolk into oil. Blend it with honey. Apply and leave on for 15 minutes before rinsing off.

A perennial favourite is the oatmeal mask. Mix one tsp of oatmeal with one tsp of milk. Leave it on face for 15 minutes and then wash it off.

Equally effective is the one made of one tsp of powdered yeast mixed with two tsp of warm water. Leave it on for 20 minutes and then wash it off with cold water.

Eye Soothers: Tea bags dipped in cold water, placed on closed eyes, or a half-inch slice of cucumber placed over eyelids while lying in bed are useful in soothing tired eyes.

For dark circles: Pat cotton wool soaked in milk under the eyes.

For a dingy neck: Mix one tsp of honey with two eggs (white). Add enough wheat bran or atta to make a paste. Beat well and rub on your neck. Leave for few minutes and wash it with warm water.

Toothpowder and mouthwashes: Use a mixture of one part table salt with two parts baking powder or add pulverized lemon and orange peel dentifrice to whiten teeth. To make a clove mouth wash, infuse three tsp of well bruised cloves in a pint of water. Boil for an hour in a covered vessel. Cool, filter and bottle.

Basic hair shampoo: Shred a cake of Pears or Castile soap in a china jar. Pour boiling water over the shreds till they are covered. Cooling will set the jelly. To condition your hair, beat an egg into two tsp of this jelly. For dry hair add one tsp of oil, coconut or olive oil, to the same measure of soap jelly. For greasy hair, substitute ½ tsp of ammonia for the oil.

Protein conditioners: This is mixture of equal proportion of gram flour, lemon juice and curd. Rub the mixture into hair. Wash with soap. Follow up with a lemon or vinegar rinse. Or take one egg, one tsp of vinegar, and two tsp of any vegetable oil. Beat together in a bowl till smooth. Massage into hair with fingertips. Wash it off with lukewarm water.

Hand lotion: Mix two tsp of lemon juice with two tsp of glycerine. Pour into a bottle and shake well before use. Stroke onto hands, working from the finger tips towards the wrist and then rub hands together as if washing up.

Nail strengthener: Mix equal quantities of castor oil and glycerine. Rub onto fingernails and cuticles.

Foot soothers: Mix one tsp curd with one tsp of powdered sugar. Rub on feet and between toes. Leave on for five minutes and then wash it off with warm water. To make a dusting powder, mix 2 tsp of powdered orrisroot, six tsp of rice powder and one tsp of powdered alum. Keep in an airtight container.

Bath salts: Use borax crystals mixed with drops of either eau de cologne, attar of rose or lavender oil.

Anti perspirant: Use equal portion of borax and starch.

Deodorant: Mix half an ounce of powdered borax, a quarter-ounce of powdered alum and juice of two alums into a litre of boiling water. Bottle it on cooling.

Natural fragrance: Take one part of herb (any fragrant one that you fancy) or flower petals, preferably rose, or your favorite spices and four parts of oil or glycerine. The longer it is kept in sun - a month for instance - the stronger the scent.

Spicy scent: Take three tsp of broken cinnamon sticks and one and a half tsp of bruised cloves and put them in a pint of alcohol. Store in a warm, dark place for a week. Shake often, strain and bottle it.

You can see for yourself what a multitude of gifts nature has for you to use!

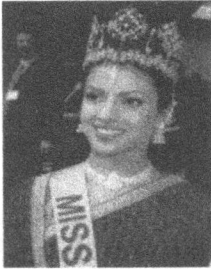

Priyanka Chopra – Miss World 2000

She was the only Indian in USA to have been selected at state level for the National Opus Honor Choir. She has done extensive charity work back in India and USA like joining the CAF and CII in their literacy programme and is their ambassador. Member of the support group for the thalassaemic children in U.P., India. Participated in the adult education awareness program with the NGOs in the peripheral areas of Bareilly. She joined the Indian Govt. sponsored Polio Eradication Programme as a volunteer, she has also helped raise funds for the destitutes at Boston, USA. That is Priyanka Chopra, Miss World 2000 for you!

For Priyanka, participating in the contest was born out of the desire to experience everything she possibly can in life. "My strong point is my adaptability, thanks to my army background," she says. Daughter of Lt. Col. Dr Ashok Chopra and Dr Madhu Chopra, she adds, "My father is a disciplinarian. He taught me the value of time management, how to conduct oneself in society, instilled in me a sense of confidence, an ease in making friends and an adaptability to any situation." She credits her mother with teaching her to be responsible for the consequences of her decisions and her younger brother for sending her photos to Femina Miss India because of his undying faith in her.

Priyanka's tips:

Teeth and oral hygiene: Cleanliness is very important. Taking calcium tablets is advisable. Consult a dentist for teeth and oral hygiene. Avoid sweets and aerated drinks. Use a recommended brand of toothpaste.

Eyes and Skin: Include lots of fresh green leafy vegetables and carrots in the diet. They contain vitamin A.

Keep eyes very clean. Practicing Yoga too helps keep eyes and skin healthy and beautiful. I use a moisturising soap and body lotion. In winter, taking oil bath and then moisturising with a moisturiser helps a lot.

For Hair: Avoid harsh chemicals. Massage with coconut oil once a week. Wash hair after every three days with suitable shampoo and use conditioner every time. Apply eggs and curd on your hair. Trim hair after every six weeks.

Diet: Regular, balanced diet helps a lot. Include fresh green leafy vegetables and fruits in your diet.

Priyanka's diet:

Morning: Vegetable juice.

Breakfast: Milk or two eggs and fruit.

Lunch: ½ cup rice, Dal, two chapattis, vegetable sabji two katoris.

Evening: Fruits.

Dinner: Salad, chicken, chappatti.

Water: Three to four litres a day.

Avoid spicy, oily food.

Exercises: Priyanka exercises at least one hour a day, especially aerobics and Yoga. She feels that meditation is very important.

This genuine, selfless, down to earth, warm and loving girl is zooming towards stardom.

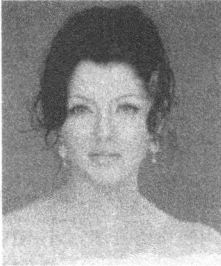

Dr. Aditi Govitrikar – Lakdawala
Mrs. World 2001

"What is unique about you?" the question was asked in the year 2001 in Las Vegas, U.S.A.

The contestant answered, "For the world though Indian I am fair and light eyed, for India I am a doctor and a model and for my family I am the only one who has bungee jumped."

The audience burst into applause and Aditi Govitrikar - Lakdawala was crowned as Mrs. World 2001. It was Mrs.World pageant and 47 countries had participated in it.

Says Aditi, "After my MBBS., one day my boyfriend, my husband now, and I were on our way to some place when I saw a hoarding inviting women to 'Enter Gladrags Super Model Contest' in June 1996. He suggested I take part in it and I won it. It was my first beauty pageant. Again, I took part in Mrs.World 2001 and I won it, too. It was quite an impulsive decision to take part in the Gladrags Super Model Contest. After that, of course, my career as a model started.

Ask Aditi about the preparations for Mrs.World pageant and she says, "There is a lot of effort that has to go in preparing for an international pageant. Unfortunately, I didn't have that kind of backing from anybody. I had to do everything on my own. Again, unfortunately I did not get much time which I wished I had. I just had 10 days in hand.

I approached Dhiren Shah, owner of Sheetal store. Luckily, he and his team designed everything for me, evening gown, clothes, my full wardrobe. To the point they even put matching bangles, earrings for me. I don't think without them it could have been possible. So that was taken care of.

For exercises and workout I got a personal trainer for eight days. Sameer Chaura was the one who trained me for those eight days. I had to wake up early and workout for one hour in the morning and then rush to work. There was no time to go to a dietician.

So that was all!"

Aditi thinks that what one needs to be successful is within yourself. If you dream, you will achieve it and if you dream big, you will achieve bigger. Positive thinking works.

Aditi's tips on personal care:

Teeth and oral hygiene: Naturally, cleanliness is crucial. Using good quality toothbrush and toothpaste is important. Regular check up with your dentist after every six months is a must. Avoid aereated drinks as they harm your teeth and inner system.

Eyes: I wear kajal and a little mascara before going out. As soon as I return home, I remove eye make-up with Clarins make-up remover. I don't forget to wear sunglasses whenever I go out in the sun.

Skin: Taking shower at least twice a day, even in winter is best for cleanliness and fresh feeling. No matter how tired you are, wash your face before you go to bed. Moisturise skin regularly. Be particular about the things that are used for makeup. Use good quality products. I go to Kaya Clinic once a month for skin polishing. So facial is not needed. Don't keep make-up on for too long. It is better to splash water on your face when the work is over. Cleansing gel is very good for removing make-up.

Manicure, pedicure etc: Regular pedicure is a must. Get it done professionally. Avoid using artificial nails. Use nail polish but don't forget to let the nails breathe once in a month for at least two days.

Hair: Oil hair once a month. Use conditioner every time after using shampoo. It is good to wash hair every third day. Due to colouring hair becomes a bit rough, so as far as possible avoid colouring them.

Aditi's diet:

Breakfast: It varies. Sometimes I eat, sometimes I skip it. Sometimes it is cornflakes with milk or upma or sevaya or eggs or dosa.

Lunch: Two to three chappattis, a bowl of vegetables, a bowl of dal. I love pickles but I eat them in small quantity.

Evening: I munch microwave popcorn, chiwda or bakarwadi while watching TV, when I am at home.

Night: Mostly I am out. I prefer Chinese or Thai Food.

I use normal sugar. I remind myself to drink a lot of water.

Aditi attributes her success to her husband and her mother-in-law. She says, "It was a very big risk that I left medicine for modelling. Everybody was against it and said that it was risky. But my husband said, "Go ahead. You can come back to medicine, whenever you want. My mother-in-law looked after my child. I didn't have to worry about it."

Special advice for mothers:

If you were fit before experiencing motherhood you should be fit as a mother, too, not for others but for yourself. I took iron and vitamin tablets that were suggested by my gynaecologist during my pregnancy. I used to drink coconut water everyday and stuck to my regular healthy food.

As for exercising, you should rest only for six weeks after the delivery. After eight weeks you can start regular workouts. Both homemakers and office-going women have a hectic schedule. But everyday you should give 10 minutes to yourself, only for yourself. That is not difficult. Go in a room. In that time if you want to be fit and you have stomach problem, do crunches. If you do 100 crunches a day, then you don't have to worry at all. Or else, in those 10 minutes you can walk, go up and down the stairs. If you are already fit, in those 10 minutes you can meditate or just listen to music or read a book. If you do that you will start feeling better. You will definitely help do better in your family life, and your professional life."

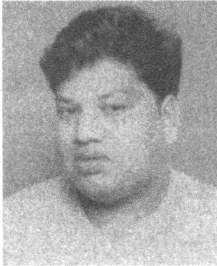

Shakir Shaikh – Choreographer

Shakir Shaikh is a well-known choreographer and a person responsible for training the male and female contestants of pageants and polishing many precious beauties.

It was since his school days that Shakir was hypnotized by the glamour, the make-up, the look and every trend of fashion. After SSC, he chose a college where he could observe a lot of glamour and fashion. Soon Shakir was choreographing dance shows for the college successfully. At one point of time he took up one fashion show for competition and they were judged as the best college in an intercollege competition. He won the best choreographer award. He began to put more efforts to do fashion shows and started taking fashion seriously. With his choreography the college won all the intercollegiate competitions at Mumbai city, Maharashtra state level and even at the national level.

Now, people started knowing about him and the college models also turned into professional models. By that time he got invited to professional shows like that of Lubna Adam and Noyonika Chatterji.

Says Shakir, "Being a fashion choreographer my job is to visualise something and go beyond others' imagination all in the aspects of lighting, designing and music.

Being a dance choreographer Shakir already had a good sense of music. After hearing the words he started choosing perfect music and that level and interest set him apart from other people in the industry because most of the choreographers depend on other music companies. He has his own bank of music. Even today, he sets up his music very differently. "Music is the soul of a fashion show. If the show goes with good music, garments work better in a somewhat dreamy and spellbound atmosphere," he says.

Shakir has seen highs and lows. There were times when he had to think that how was he going to survive, but there were also times where on the basis of one show he received at least a dozen offers! Shakir has worked with winners of Miss India contests like Ujwala Raut, Netra Raghuraman, Carol Gracias and Karishma Modi. One of the biggest shows that he has done has been the Shaina N.C. show before which Shaina had told him, "Shakir, we either make it or break it. If you don't do my show well, I don't know you; or else you do all my shows." He has worked with her over and over again.

He has done a detailed study of the psychological presentation of the models in India. "You have to take care while working with fresh models as well as with professional models," he says. "How to keep your head cool, be calm, how not to lose head are the things to think over. The work has to be with smooth mental pressure, not with hard mental torture. Of course the mental pressure has to be on the model to give the delivery but has to be so smooth that they deliver it with joy and not with force. If they are scared, they come on stage and make mistakes and again get scared that they may get shouting from their "choreographer." He had been handling Super Model pageant, Miss Mumbai pageant and lot many successfully when he was offered yet another challenge. It was the Miss Lashkara show. He had to handle typical Indian beauties from small towns who were unaware of fashion trends. The job set to him was to train those girls as perfectly trained models on stage. After the 15th day, the girls were as confident as any other model from Mumbai. Then onwards he handles Miss Lashkara every year. Says he, "I wish more and more serious people come into fashion and take this profession seriously. Make the best out of it in terms of business and there is a lot of potential in terms of money. I forsee lot of growth."

Miss India Worldwide Pageant: Brief Introduction

Miss India Worldwide Pageant is organised by the New York-based India Festival Committee, a non-profit, voluntary organisation established in 1974. India Festival Committee is a pioneer in conducting Indian Pageants and fashion shows in USA and worldwide, and has been conducting Miss India New York, and Miss India USA Pageants since 1980.

The name Miss India Worldwide was registered under the trademark act of USA and has been granted the Trademark by the commissioner of Patents and Trademark of the United States Government.

Mr Dharmatma Saran, founder and chairman of the Indian Festival Committee, in 1990 decided to take the pageant one step further to an international level and initiated the Miss India Worldwide Pageant. For the first time ever, Asian Indian communities from all over the world came together in New York for this event.

The pageant was an instant success and was acclaimed as "The most glamorous Indian function in the world." Miss India Worldwide is organised in various parts of the world. To celebrate India's 50th Independence Day, the pageant was organised in Mumbai in 1997. In the year 1998, the exotic and beautiful city of Singapore was chosen as the venue.

Winners of Miss India contests throughout the world (e.g. Miss India UK/Miss India Singapore) can participate in this contest. The contestants in all the pageants are of Indian origins, (either of their parents should be Indian), unmarried in the age group of 17-27 years of age and should be citizens, residents and/or born in the country which they represent.

The India Festival Committee selects distinguished local organisations in various parts of the world by advertising in the newspapers to conduct national pageants in their respective countries.

The pageant consists of four segments: Evening Gown, Indian Dress, Talent and Question & Answers. The winners of all the various national pageants from all over the world vie for this glamorous and prestigious title of Miss India Worldwide. The winner of the contest is then crowned with the title of 'Miss Worldwide'.

The India Festival Committee motivates and guides its winners and contestants to take up charity causes.

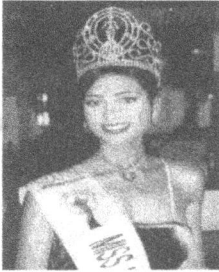

Melissa Bhagat –
Miss Teen Toronto '95,
Miss India Canada '98,
Miss India Worldwide '99,
Miss Canada '99 Runner up-1,
Miss Millennium Girl '99-2000

Melissa was always fond of India and she made it a point to collect more and more information about India and Indians. Born and brought up in Toronto she says, "Though I don't live in India, I love India a lot. I have very positive emotions towards India and for Indians." Melissa was Miss Toronto '95 and then Miss India Canada '98.

Melissa points out that her parents have played an integral role in her successful career. A graduate in international relations, Melissa has mastered French and English language. In fact, at a very young age, Melissa was enrolled in dancing, acting and modelling classes. She has done a course in Jazz, Ballet, Tap, Acrobatics, Hip-hop and Salsa dance and loves travelling and cooking. For the past years Melissa has been travelling across the world as a role model promoting unity in diversity among the international Indian communities.

She has been actively involved in noble charity causes of the likes of: Mother Theresa's Missionaries of Charity (India), Nargis Dutt Cancer Foundation (New York, USA), Sick Kids Children's Hospital (Toronto, Canada), Safe City Program (Brampton, Canada) and Canadian Heart & Stroke Foundation (Canada).

Melissa admits that though she is involved in charitable causes her favourite is 'World Vision International' and has so become the official South Asian spokesperson for their Canadian organisation. She had also organised a golf tournament in Canada for raising funds to help women and children in India. Titled as 'The Hope of India' the event was a grand success.

Being Miss-Millennium and the 'Face of Tourism', she has travelled across the globe focusing on core issues. In fact, she hopes to continue her efforts and intends to pursue a career in International Politics as ambassador in foreign affairs.

Melissa attributes her success to her confidence, intelligence and inner beauty as opposed to her physical attributes. She says, "I'm not a supermodel, and I'm not perfect."

Melissa's beauty tips:

Dental & oral hygiene: Melissa brushes her teeth with American Toothpaste thrice a day and gargles her mouth after every meal. Many a times for the sake of exercise (for jaws and teeth) she consumes whole fruits by chewing them properly and eats sugar-free chewing gum.

Eyes: Keeps slice of cucumber on eyelids while sleeping. Avoids undue stress on eyes. Uses sunglasses while moving out to protect eyes from sunrays. Consumes food rich in vitamin-A and has green vegetables and ample fruits. Every day she drinks two glasses of carrot juice and eats two bowls of leafy vegetables.

Hair: Washes her hair with shampoo twice a week. Uses a comb with thick and wide bristles. Combs her hair regularly during the day. Massages her scalp with olive and almond oil once in a month. Applies egg and then washes it off with lukewarm water. She has never had dandruff problem.

Skin: Keeps herself clean and washes face with a lot of water at least thrice a day. Uses apricot scrub (twice a week) for cleaning it properly and then applies oil-free moisturiser to the face and neck. Always removes make-up by using oil-free moisturising cleanser. Before sleeping at night applies vitamin E night cream to face and neck. She eats lots of fruits, green vegetables, and drinks a lot of water. Avoids cold drinks, aerated drinks and oily foods to keep her skin glowing.

During the day she prefers natural look—just uses lot of mascara and lip balm or lip-gloss. For evening/night she simply adds foundation and eyeliner. She doesn't use foundation unless she is working.

Once a month she visits a beauty parlour and gets her face clean. She suggests body massages with olive oil twice a month. She is highly influenced by Mickey Mehta and has stopped non-veg food and dairy products.

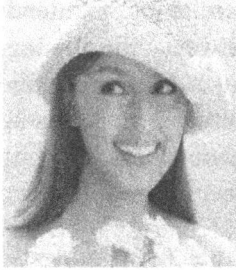

Aarti Chhabria – Miss Millennium, Miss Worldwide 1999

Slim, beautiful and energetic, Aarti was barely 17 years old, and in fact, the youngest contestant in the India Queen Beauty Pageant '99. It so happened that Aarti had bagged the title Giant's Pageant, at the tender age of 15, and one of the organisers of the India Queen Beauty Pageant, who was present at the contest, met Aarti, complimented her and suggested her to participate in the India Queen Beauty Pageant.

Aarti, witty and beautiful as she is, could easily make it and won the title. She also won awards in the various categories like Best Complexion, Best Smile and Best Eyes. Aarti had then to prepare herself for the Miss India Worldwide contest to be held at New Jersey, America. The contest was on November 26, 1999. Aarti won the Miss India Worldwide title, but as the contest was held in November, she was crowned as 'Miss India Worldwide, 2000'.

During the contest as rounds progressed, beauty took the back seat and the focus shifted to intelligence and presence of mind. The final question was, "What should be the role of the woman of the millennium?' and on the spur of the moment Aarti answered, "The woman of the millennium should be self confident, beautiful, intelligent, having the go-getter/winning attitude, and should spread the message of love, integrity and be able to safeguard Indian human values."

Aarti recalls she could make it because she had prepared for it, she specifically developed the habit of reading newspapers and watching TV news. She says, "I hated reading but just to gain confidence, I started reading books and it helped me a lot. Also one has to keep oneself updated on all the different subjects and the current happenings all over." And just because she had read much on politics she could answer the questions asked.

Aarti was keen to participate in the Femina Miss India contest but couldn't, as conventionally Aarti is not so tall. She is just 5.5" as against the required height of 5.7" for the Femina Miss India Contest. She was also called for Miss India USA as the judge and has also received 'Glamour' award during the Millennium Bollywood awards.

Aarti's beauty secrets:

Dental & oral hygiene: Consume vegetables like carrot, radish that require proper chewing and gargle after every meal. By eating carrots her skin, eyes and hair have become excellent. Use a branded toothpaste.. Avoid aerated drinks as they form a yellow layer on your teeth. Do mouth exercise like stretching. Practice clear diction, it boosts your self-confidence. Speak clearly, do not mumble. This too shows your confidence level.

Eyes: Maintain eyebrows regularly at least once in fortnight by removing extra hair than shaping eyebrows. Use eyeliner and mascara of reputed companies. Always take a trial before using them. Use sunglasses while moving out. In case of dark circles, keep a slice of cucumber/wet cotton strips on eyelids. If eyes are too strained then keep cold napkin or ice cubes on eyes while sleeping. To make eyelids look thick apply castor oil on eyelids. Avoid sleeping in the afternoon.

Face: It is advisable to apply the mixture of Adapalene and Eumusome in case you get pimples. For blackheads, keep your face clean. Also take a face-clean-up (take steam before a face-clean-up) and then rub a piece of ice and apply a moisturiser. Do not use soap but use a face wash at least three to four times a day to keep your face clean. Use baby oil while cleaning/removing make-up. It is always advisable to massage your body with baby oil before having a bath.

Palms, feet and nails: Keep arms and legs clean by waxing them regularly. It is advisable to get pedicure and manicure done regularly too. Use a suitable hand and body lotion of a reputed company. Keep nails clean as they reflect your personality. Keep nails in lukewarm water mixed with lemon and then massage them with a cream or oil. Never use artificial nails. Keep nails of suitable length so that one can always file them properly.

Hair: Massage hair and scalp with castor oil mixed with coconut oil; this also helps avoid dandruff, untimely discoloration and hair loss. Do not leave the oil overnight; wash it off after two hours. Use amla powder for hair. Wash hair with shampoo and use hair conditioner to keep them soft and shining. Cut the ends of hair at least once in three months.

Diet: Spinach is a must in your every day meal. Eat lots of carrot, beetroot, lettuce, cabbage with some lemon juice and salt before every meal. Design your diet programme for one month. You can be flexible in your lunch/dinner but see to it that you have the entire foodstuff as mentioned in your diet program. Eat fresh vegetables and have proper food. Do not eat preserved food/ vegetables. Have one glass of milk in the morning and have chopped fruits, especially apple and lemon juice, for breakfast. In the evening at around 5 o'clock eat fruits and have some buttermilk. Support your diet with vitamin capsules.

Avoid potato, rice, ice creams, sweets, wafers, oily and junk food and aerated drinks. Eat non-veg food once in a while, but in a limited quantity.

Exercise: Exercise everyday at least for one hour. Crunches are very effective for stomach.

Pointers for winning:

A beautiful woman/girl should be beautiful in all aspects. She should be intelligent and impressive. Beauty means equilibrium—a balance between face, body, personality, clean heart and physical beauty. Beauty originates from the heart. Such women always appear fresh and have beautiful and expressive eyes. A woman should be able to express herself freely, she should be convincing, affectionate, kind and should have a good dressing sense.

Crunches for stomach:

Lie down on your back. Bend your legs. Ask someone to stand on your feet and then get up lifting your back.

Lie down on your back. Arms folded under your head. Then do crunches for either side, first the left, then the right side. Do it gently. Repeat for 50 counts.

For lower stomach: Lie down on your back. Arms folded under your head. Lift your legs at 90 degrees. Cross your legs and bend in knees. Then do the crunches (Aarti does this for 50 counts daily.)

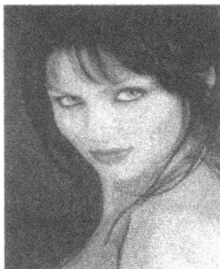

Yana Gupta – Model

Yana has been one beauty queen born and brought up in Czech Republic but settled in India after marriage. She loves living in India. Her interest in spirituality has taken her all over India on vacations, mostly in meditation camps.

She came to India more than three years back and has been working as a model. Says she, "One of my close friends was very keen on this profession. She started telling me about models and the fashion world. As a fan, I had practiced ramp walking in her house. We were 14 at that time!

At 15 we joined a one-month course run by an advertising agency. The company selected me as a model and I started working with them. Soon they sent me to Prague, the capital of Czech Republic. There were many modelling agencies around and much more happening. The agency used to send me abroad. I started travelling regularly to Europe, USA, Japan learning more about international fashion. Modelling in India was a chance affair which just happened.

Yana's tips for aspiring models:

Be a professional, always be on time, always try to learn, try to enjoy whatever job you are doing otherwise don't do it. Have an open mind for learning and experiencing new things. Forget about your ego or pride whenever people ask you to do certain things.

Just follow optimistically. Unfortunately modelling is more about the creativity of the people around you, the agencies, photographers, designers, thats the reason I switched over to movies where I could bring my creativity to the fore. You have to go with their flow and cooperate with them. We should develop the art to be successful in this creative field.

Tips for being healthy:

Dental & oral hygiene: A very high level of cleanliness is crucial.

Eyes: Clean eyes from inside before going to bed with the help of cotton buds dipped in lens solution. Wash eyes with pure water. Whenever tired, put cucumber slices on eyes.

Eyebrows: Shape eyebrows once in four months.

Skin: Moisturising face and hands regularly is advisable. Moisturise whole body once a week. Get massage once a week. Clean-up after every sauna or steam bath is very effective. After the bath you can easily remove blackheads with slight pressure.

Mix yoghurt, honey and carrot or just honey and massage your face. Leave it on face and then wash it out. This is the best face pack. Never use soap for face. Herbal soap-free face wash is beneficial for washing face.

Feet & soles: Mud therapy is good for skin. Never forget to clean feet and soles thoroughly.

Hair: As I sweat while exercising, I shampoo and condition hair every day. Oiling and massaging hair once a week is very good. Massaging activates the skin on scalp. Trim hair once in two months.

Diet: It is better to eat five to six times a day, small portions each time rather than big ones. Eat healthy food, lots of vegetables, fruits and drink lots of fresh vegetable and fruit juices. One could also eat salads, pieces of vegetables, like capsicum or fruits as snacks. Eating at same and right times is very important. Oil is very important and you need it. You should use proper kind of oil. I use olive oil. Oil provides vitamin A and Vitamin E. Drinking coconut water every day is the best as it is very natural, tamper-free and best for body.

Avoid drinking tea, coffee, soft drinks. Instead drink green tea or decafinated tea.

Exercises: Working out six times a week is very effective. Exercises are very important, so is Yoga and taking long walks. Yana has experimented with different different forms of exercises like Yoga, Taichi, swimming, boating, tracking and so on.

Yalta's exercise schedule:

Day 1: Upper part with weights

Day 2: Cardio

Day 3: Lower part with weights

Day 4: Cardio

So in this way I do cardio exercises alternate day and I take rest once in a week.

Till now we have been talking about beauty, and various tips for maintaining it, even we've had experts sharing their line of action and methods, and also we've had models sharing their experiences with us.

In the previous chapters, we have discussed in-depth the theme of beauty-tips for maintaining it, advice from the experts such as healthcare professionals, models and those in the field of fashion, glamour and beauty care.

If you too would like to develop your personality, then there is a place just right for you; where under expert guidance you can cultivate beauty, grace and poise. And who knows, you could be the next Miss India?!!

Dynamic Beauty and Personality Development Institute

Founded by Mrs. Jayashree Pathak, the Dynamic Beauty and Personality Development Institute provides a course in Beauty and Personality Development. The course is categorised into basic and advance. The basic course consists of seven integrated modules which helps to develop oneself as a perfect individual with a sound personality. Wherein apart from looking good, one can learn various other aspects of beauty, as beauty without brains is incomplete. The advance course is meant for specialisation wherein one can discover various opportunities ahead in the glamour world of modelling, beauty contests, films etc. Any individual above the age of 10 years is eligible for the course.

The first module is an introduction to perfect style, and training in areas like facing the camera, correct postures, ramp walking etc.

The second module includes a systematic programme on fitness, nutrition, diet and exercise, while the third module consists of personality development, diction, conversational skills and etiquette.

The fourth module focusses on hair dos, pinning, using rollers, etc. that would improve the looks.

The fifth module includes make-up and touch-over techniques that could enhance ones personality and make one look attractive.

Skin care, hair care and eye care is included in the sixth module that provides information and preventive measures that can help maintain one's looks.

Last but not the least is the seventh module that focuses on smile and oral hygiene. This involves smiling techniques and smiling exercises that give you a perfect smile, whereas, the advance course provides specialisation in any one subject of the learner's interest like modelling, participating in beauty contest, film/TV serials/ theatre etc.

The institute has to its credit many models who represent the dynamic new generation.

There are also those who have only done the basic course as a matter of interest and find it helpful in their personal lives.

For further information, contact:

Mrs. Jayashree Pathak,
17/393, Vijaynagar Hsg. Society,
S.N. Road, Andheri (E),
Mumbai - 400 069
Tel: 26823095
Mobile: 9323710920